A Charge Nurse's Guide:

Navigating the Path of Leadership
2nd Edition

Cathy Leary, R.N. & Scott J. Allen, Ph.D.

Center for Leader Development Press
Cleveland, Ohio
www.centerforleaderdevelopment.com

A Charge Nurse's Guide
Navigating the Path of Leadership

Center for Leader Development Press
Cleveland, Ohio
www.centerforleaderdevelopment.com
cathyleary1@netscape.net
scott@cldmail.com

Leary, Cathy, 1943-
Allen, Scott, 1972-

ISBN: 0-9773726-1-8
Library of Congress Control Number: 2005934073

First Edition, 2006
Second Edition, 2014
Printed in USA

Cover Design: Andy Shive

Production: Bookmasters, Ashland, Ohio 44805

Acknowledgements

The authors would like to thank the following individuals for their thoughtful contribution in the form of feedback, editing and encouragement.

Jessica Allen
Catherine Anson
Lisa Aurilio, R.N.
D. Barry, R.N.
Stephen B. Becker
Louise and Bill Bradley
Julie Byrne, R.N.
Lynn Cheslock, R.N.
L. Martin Cobb
Valerie L. DeCamp, R.N.
Lisa Deptowicz, R.N.
Martha Duffy, R.N.
Nancy Haas, R.N.
Cathy L. Hadley-Samia, R.N.
Debbie Hawk, R.N.
Antoinette Kelley, R.N.
Unhee Kim, R.N.
Curtis Leary
Suzanne M. Gill, R.N.
Sarah McManus, R.N.
Thomas C. Olver
Cam Ray, R.N.
Evelyn C. Samples, R.N.
Denise Saraviti, R.N.
Lee Ann Schaffert, R.N.
Andy Shive
Amelia Smith, R.N.

Dedications

Cathy

To my husband, Curtis Leary, whose love and generous spirit
sustain me.

Scott

To my wife Jessica.

"Love does not consist in gazing at each other but in looking
together in the same direction."
—Antoine de Saint-Exupery

To all nurses everywhere.

Just before his death in 1963, the great American poet Robert Frost wrote his last poem to his nurse, Janet Forbes:

"I met you on a cloudy and dark day and when you smiled and spoke the room was filled with sunshine. The way you smiled at me has given my heart a change of mood and saved some part of a day I had rued."

A Charge Nurse's Guide

Navigating the Path of Leadership

Table of Contents

Preface

This brief but important book is designed to augment your leadership education and experience. It is also designed for a busy clinician who does not have the time or energy to wade through hundreds of pages of text. This book can be read quickly in one two-hour sitting or as you have 10-15 minutes here and there.

In conceiving this book, our goal was to develop a simple but comprehensive guide that is focused on the most crucial information you need to lead effectively in your role as charge nurse. As a result, we have focused on topics such as leadership, stakeholders/resources, self-awareness, patient safety, delegation, leading through conflict, navigating change and mentoring. We have devoted separate chapters to patient satisfaction and patient safety. These are over-arching concepts that require the implementation of all leadership skills.

Each chapter is divided into two primary sections: **Personal Lessons** and **Resources & References**. The Personal Lessons sections may contain: our thoughts on the topic, reflections, things to remember, and case studies. The Resources & References sections may include: short articles by other authors, key terms/acronyms, additional resources and references.

We welcome your feedback and wish you all the best as you navigate the path of leadership…

Chapter One
Me? A Leader?

Yes, you are a leader! As a charge nurse, you are in a key role to make health care work for everyone—patients, families, physicians, nurses and the many other people who are involved in the care and healing of patients. The word that may be unexpected is *leader.* You probably did not sign up to be a leader when you decided to become a registered nurse. *Caregiver* might have been the descriptive word you had in mind—and that you are. Caregiving is the essence of nursing. However, if you think about it, much of being a great charge nurse has to do with being a great leader. A great charge nurse leads a healthcare team and its individuals to manage the care of patients efficiently and effectively. Leadership is the key to transforming a group of individuals into a high functioning team. Under great leadership, the team will perform the many tasks and responsibilities required for patient care and a great leader can transform a list of tasks into a coordinated and energizing approach to healing.

"You gain strength, courage and confidence by every experience in which you really stop to look fear in the face. You must do the thing you think you cannot do."—Eleanor Roosevelt, author and 32nd First Lady of the United States

A Balancing Act

As you know, a nurse must perform a skillful balancing act each day. You are responsible for many aspects of care as well as other duties—managing patients' medications, treatments, activities of daily living, and information; documenting the status and care given to patients; coordinating the schedules of diagnostic and treatment procedures handled by other departments; orienting new employees; and, of course, managing your time so that you can accomplish everything in the hours allotted. *This balancing act is one of the most important things to learn.* It can be overwhelming and, at first, may even seem impossible. Leadership of a nursing team is difficult because you are responsible not merely for one patient, but many. Nothing remains static.

Things are changing all around you—admissions, discharges, patient status, unexpected demands and so forth. To be effective, you must depend upon your colleagues to work as a team. Often, this is the most challenging aspect of your job. Everyone is "doing their own thing" as each person has an assigned role of individual responsibilities. To add to the challenge, some people prefer to work on their own and have little natural inclination to be part of a team.

An additional complicating factor is that some days you are in a formal leadership role and others not. Sometimes, you are the one asking for help from your colleagues. Other times, you are part of a team that is led by someone else. You are both leader and follower and required to serve both roles well.

"Leaders are people who do the right thing; managers are people who do things right. Both roles are crucial, and they differ profoundly. I often observe people in top positions doing the wrong things well."—*Warren Bennis, leadership author*

As charge nurse, you are the first line of leadership in your organization. You have the responsibility to help everyone better serve patients, to help one another, and to help the mission of your organization—what an exciting and crucial position. If you fully embrace and succeed in this role, it is certain to be one of your greatest accomplishments.

"Leadership should be born out of the understanding of the needs of those who will be affected by it."—*Marion Anderson, contralto vocalist*

A Difficult Role

If you have served as a charge nurse before, you know there are many days when you go home thinking, "This is too much." That is a natural feeling. Your role is to meet the needs of a number of stakeholders, and those needs often feel insatiable. You simply cannot do everything for every person. Since you have chosen to be a nurse, you may have a natural desire to please and serve others. Learning how to be an effective leader will help you to balance this goal with the sometimes-overwhelming demands of your many stakeholders. Few professions are as demanding and difficult as nursing; however, it is also the noblest of professions because *you make a difference in the lives of others*. Remember this when you have a discouraging thought—it will help you to return to your true mission.

"The only real training for leadership is leadership." —*Anthony Jay, leadership author*

People and Systems

In your role as charge nurse, your assignment is to manage the work systems and processes of the healthcare organization on behalf of the patients. However, the most precious asset of the healthcare organization is its people. Every hand, heart and mind is required to accomplish what needs to be done and an effective charge nurse is the key to joining these two ingredients—the people *and* the work systems.

Often nurses are assigned to the role of charge nurse without adequate preparation. The decision may be made based on tenure or clinical excellence, not because of demonstration of leadership skills. Being inadequately prepared for the role of charge nurse may cause you to feel dissatisfaction. Effective functioning as a leader is difficult even with experience and preparation. It can be doubly so without the benefit of a leadership development program. Of course there are mentors, classes, observations and other opportunities for training but these often focus on the systems (e.g., electronic medical records, equipment, work-flow) and rarely prepare you for the "people" part of the role.

The truth is, of course, that you learn on the job. While scary and even a little risky, this can be an effective way to learn. No class and no mentoring can *fully* prepare you for the role of charge nurse because every day and every patient is different. No matter how long you serve in this role, you will continually learn as you go. You will be amazed at how often you are faced with new challenges. The most effective approach is to get a firm grip on the basics, and your confidence will grow as you progress. A nurse is in a unique position to understand how the systems and departments of a healthcare organization work. As charge nurse your challenge is to mesh this knowledge with the needs of the patients and the potential of the team.

"Effective leadership is putting first things first. Effective management is discipline, carrying it out."—*Stephen Covey, leadership author*

Using Your Resources

It is assumed that your clinical knowledge, patient assessment skills, ability to help physicians at the bedside and other aspects of the clinical role of nurses are solidly in place. In addition to being a resource for the clinical aspects of nursing care, you are also required to lead the team. This may feel daunting. However, it is rare for nurses to feel they are "ready" to be in charge. If you are assigned to learn the role of charge nurse, embrace it and go for it. Someone thinks you are ready, even if you don't. Chances are you will thrive in the role. Never forget that you are surrounded by people who can help you. This does not mean that every day you should say, "I need help. I can't do all this work." It means that when you are in the rare situation of feeling truly overwhelmed, you can reach out and ask others for help, guidance or advice. Get in the habit of helping others and they will be delighted to help you when you ask for assistance.

"We are not independent, but interdependent."—*Buddha, spiritual leader, 560-480 BC*

Leading the Team

A genuine passion for working with people is one of the most important assets you can bring to the role of charge nurse. Most nurses want to feel a part of a team, and gain joy from helping others. *Displaying true appreciation toward others for their unique gifts is a large part of being an effective charge nurse.* This simple concept is difficult to teach because it stems from an inherent zeal for health care and for working with a team of colleagues.

If you embrace this challenge and give it your best shot, you will be amazed at the results. Being an effective charge nurse requires you to use your clinical knowledge, emotional intelligence, social skills and technical expertise. You will accomplish more than you ever thought possible, and you will feel fulfilled, frustrated, tired and elated. However, we look forward to the day when you hear the following from a colleague—"The day always goes better when you are in charge."

"Not everyone can be good at both leading and managing. Some people have the capacity to become excellent managers but not strong leaders. Others have great leadership potential but have great difficulty becoming strong managers. Smart companies value both kinds of people and work hard to make them a part of the team." — *John P. Kotter, author*

Personal Lessons

Reflections

Reflect on your favorite supervisor
- What are the qualities that make this person a great leader?
- What specific personal attributes help this supervisor connect with others?
- Which of the quotes in this chapter would best describe this person's approach to work?

Reflect upon your thoughts of being in a leadership role
- What strengths and potential areas of weakness do you recognize in yourself? How will you manage personal areas that need improvement?
- What excites you about the charge nurse role?

- What worries you about taking on the role of charge nurse?
- What resources exist to support you as you grow and develop?
- What individuals can you rely on for positive and constructive feedback?
- What does your supervisor expect of you?

Questions for Your Supervisor

- What do I need to know about working for you? What are your expectations?
- How will you define success in this role? What goals should I have?
- What are the five most important areas of focus for a charge nurse?
- How should I approach my role with other team members on the unit/in the department?
- Are there any special skills I need to perform my job? Based on what you know of me, do you feel there is anything I need to improve to be more effective? Are there classes I can take to learn new skills?
- What will my probationary period entail? How long will it be? Who will be my mentor? How often will I get feedback on my performance?
- What are our unit goals? What is my role in helping us achieve these?
- What are the traits/behaviors of successful charge nurses on this unit?

Things to Remember

- As a charge nurse, you are in a key role to make health care work for everyone—patients, families, physicians, nurses and all the many other people who are involved in the care and healing of patients.
- An effective charge nurse successfully leads people *and* manages work systems. A charge nurse plays one of the most important roles in a healthcare organization.

- No class or mentoring will fully prepare you as charge nurse because every day and every patient is different. No matter how long you serve in this role, you will learn.
- Reflect often. Adults grow and learn through reflection. How did you do today? What could you have done better? When you stop asking these questions, you stop growing.
- Be sure you and your supervisor are on the same page. Asking the questions listed in this chapter may help you set up clear baseline expectations.
- You know you are on the right track when someone says, "The day always goes better when you are in charge."

Resources & References

Terms & Acronyms

- **Barriers/Roadblocks**—You face a number of barriers each day. These are problems that stop you from doing your job successfully. They often arise from communication problems or inadequate systems. Part of your job is to recognize these barriers and roadblocks and do your best to remove them for the team.
- **Caregiver**—This is a licensed person who provides direct care, help and protection to someone. A caregiver helps to identify, treat or prevent illness or disability.
- **Leadership**—This term is the heart of this book and is about influencing a group of people toward a common goal, which in this case, is to provide excellent care.
- **Management**—The act or art of managing; the manner of treating, directing, carrying on, or using for a purpose; conduct; administration; guidance; control; (*Webster's Revised Unabridged Dictionary*).
- **Mission Statement**—A public statement of an organization or group's purpose or reason for existence.
- **Multi-tasking**—Having many balls in the air at one time! As your responsibility in the organization increases so does the complexity of your work. Doctors, patients, co-

workers, supervisors, and others will look to you to keep several balls in the air at one time.

- **Personal Mission**—a pre-established and often self-imposed objective or purpose.
- **System**—The *American Heritage Dictionary* defines *system* as "a group of interacting, interrelated, or interdependent elements forming a complex whole." We are surrounded by systems every day. Restaurants have a system for getting your food to you in a timely manner. Likewise, your medical center has a system for efficiently admitting, treating, and discharging patients. When patient care is not efficient or if your fries are cold when they arrive, there is a systems problem. Finding and eliminating the root of systems problems is a part of your job.

Chapter Two
Leadership

Leadership defined in one word would be "influence." If you step back and think about it, we all practice the art of influence on a daily basis. This happens in your home (with your spouse/children) in the workplace (with your peers, supervisor, patients and their families) and at other institutions (e.g., places of worship, community organizations).

If you are assigned to the role of charge nurse, you have responsibility for leading a team. In this instance, you have a formal position of authority or we could also call it a formal leadership role. However, as we have discussed, each one of us (including your CEO) moves in and out of the leader/follower role. For instance, there are probably shifts when you are a follower and someone else is the charge nurse or team leader. The fluid nature of health care adds to the complexity of leading well. It is important to note that you do not need a formal title to influence or lead. In fact, leadership may occur in brief moments as when you influence your peers or a family on your unit. In essence, leaders have the ability to influence others without the use of authority. As a charge nurse you have the opportunity to practice influencing others.

So what is leadership? What makes a leader effective or ineffective? In our experience we have found that when people talk about leaders, they usually enter the conversation in one of five places: personal attributes, purpose, process, product or principles. It's likely that you judge your supervisor on some combination of these. More important, these are the criteria upon which you will be judged when serving as a leader. We call these the Five Ps.

The first P is *personal attributes*. Think of your current supervisor. Do you personally like him or her? Is he or she a nice person? Is he intelligent, achievement-oriented, empathetic, and optimistic? Does she display emotional intelligence and first-rate conflict management skills? Is he or she technically competent and self-aware? These are examples of personal attributes of an individual. If you answered "yes" to the questions above, it's likely you think well of your current supervisor. However, we all know what it feels like when this is not the case. A fundamental attribute of effective leaders is the ability to develop relationships in order to work well with others.

The second P is *purpose*, which answers the question, "Leadership for what?" Leaders are clearly aligned around a cause or purpose and influence others to follow. At times this purpose is altruistic, mission-driven and easy for others to follow. On the downside, the purpose can be self-centered, overly political and difficult to support. In healthcare, the purpose is fairly clear—patients first. Leaders with the ability to keep this purpose front and center have a very clear "north star" when faced with the many challenges inherent in healthcare. A fundamental attribute of effective leaders is setting direction and inspiring others to come along.

The third P is *process*, which describes how the leader achieves *purpose*. In other words, moving the group, organization or community from point A to point Z. By many accounts Steve Jobs of Apple used a coercive and autocratic style of moving his team toward the vision. It was *his* vision. Others may choose to use a more democratic process and highly value the involvement and "voice" of others. We would imagine you have worked for men and women at both ends of the spectrum and while all styles have an appropriate time and place, a coercive style is, in general, not found to be an inspiring approach in the long run. Thus, a fundamental attribute of effective leaders is the ability to use the appropriate leadership style for the context.

The fourth P is *product,* which is all about results. Some wonder if the success or failure of the leader can be determined prior to knowing the final results of the purpose. In other words, was the objective achieved? Was the transformation successful? Was the patient cured or did the procedure go well? These are all examples of an end product. Organizations need men and women who can successfully navigate the roadblocks, politics, and red tape, and ultimately "win." A fundamental attribute of effective leaders is the ability to achieve results even in the face of the challenges inherent in complex organizations.

"You gain credibility and authority in your career by demonstrating your capacity to take other people's problems off their shoulders and give them back solutions." — *Ronald Heifetz, leadership author*

The fifth P is *principled.* A principled leader is one who acts in accordance with morality, is honorable and demonstrates recognition of right and wrong. While it may be argued that this could be a *personal attribute*, we feel that this attribute needs specific attention. In the long run, leaders model ethical behavior and walk their talk. Trust is a fundamental tenant of any human relationship, and leaders who struggle to model the way will be limited in their ability to truly win the hearts and minds of those who follow. A fundamental attribute of effective leaders is their ability to remain principled and focused on ethical behavior.

"Nearly all men can stand adversity, but if you want to test a man's character, give him power." — *Abraham Lincoln, 16th President of the United States*

Common Sense *and* Practice

Most of what is said in this chapter is either common sense or knowledge you have acquired through life's lessons. If asked to list the characteristics of an effective leader, you would identify an excellent profile as we have above. However, common sense does not equal common practice. For example, we have all seen illustrations of slippage of good intentions in failed dieting attempts, inconsistent parenting and, unfortunately, ineffective leadership.

Putting the above-mentioned attributes into action will take deliberate practice. The good news is you have a wonderful practice field (your organization). The difficult news is that you are your own best coach and you need to prioritize the work of practicing leadership.

As a charge nurse, you will sometimes find it difficult to maintain professional and appropriate behavior. There will be interruptions and unplanned events that are disruptive to the work plan that you are attempting to accomplish. You will feel stressed and hurried. In these moments, it is easy to *react* to disconcerting circumstances in a way that diminishes your power and effectiveness as a leader.

It is important to maintain an appropriate demeanor at all times. One technique is to imagine that you are in a play and the character you are playing consistently behaves in a positive, professional manner. When you are new to leadership, this approach may help you to distance yourself a bit from personally challenging circumstances. It may help you to remember how to "act" until it becomes second nature.

"Related to leadership is the concept of power; the potential to influence. There are two kinds of power: position and personal." — *Peter Northouse, leadership author*

Practice Reflection

Even if you can recite the attributes of a good leader (The 5 Ps) and are effective in the charge nurse role, it is a good idea to give some thought to your own strengths and developmental needs. At the end of a shift it is a good habit to review the day and think about what went well, what did not, and the role *you* had in producing these outcomes. What did you do that was effective? What did you do that was ineffective? What did you do that had a positive impact on the care of the patients? What did you do to promote teamwork? What did you do to bring out the best in each individual? What would you do and say differently?

Once when I (Cathy) was doing rounds on the night shift, a new charge nurse said to me, "Do we have a policy that mandates people to respect the charge nurse? I don't think these people respect me, and I want to show them in writing where it says that they have to because I am in charge." I understood what she meant. I have been there. Taking charge on the night shift can be pretty difficult and lonely, especially when you have relatively short tenure and it feels like everyone else on duty has been working the night shift for years. If the new charge nurse assumes the demeanor of dictator, it turns into an unfortunate situation and everyone "hunkers down" to watch him or her flounder. I am sure you have seen this in your own organization. This happens, in part, because the charge nurse is unsure of his or her role. He or she is a little frightened and thinking more about herself than about how the team is doing. It can be easy to forget how it feels to be a follower or member of the team. It is important to remember that respect is *earned* not mandated.

"In organizations, real power and energy is generated through relationships. The patterns of relationships and the capacities to form them are more important than tasks, functions, roles, and positions." — *Margaret Wheatley, leadership author*

Practice Serving Others

It may be helpful to become familiar with the work of Robert K. Greenleaf, who has written on the concept of *servant leadership.* This philosophy fits quite naturally into the work of nurses. Nurses have chosen a profession of service and understand what it means to serve others. In their daily work, however, nurses are also called upon to lead. It is easy for nurses to grasp the concept of a leader as the servant of the followers. The servant leader acts as a guide for a team. Likewise, the charge nurse guides the healthcare team to accomplish all that needs to be done by serving the needs of the team. Although it may seem subtle and vague at first, servant leadership is far more effective than a top-down coercive style.

Effective charge nurses are known by their peers as good team members, trusted colleagues and hard workers. They are respectful of others and have earned the respect of peers in the role of followers. Respect must be *earned*, and it starts by respecting others. Once you have earned respect, teammates grant you the power needed to lead effectively. Therefore, the seeds for being an effective charge nurse have already been sown by the time you assume the role.

"All leaders are actual or potential power holders, but not all power holders are leaders." — *James MacGregor Burns, leadership author*

Practice Leadership

In this short introduction to the topic of leadership we have communicated that it is a complex topic. It requires you to be self-aware, balanced, strong, kind and positive. It works best when you care deeply about the patients and those who care for the patients. Leadership is a big job, and it is a wonderful, fulfilling job. One of the most important behaviors you can contribute to the work of the team is your optimism and your willingness to provide positive feedback and affirmation. This communicates to the team and its members that you trust and believe in them. Optimism and a positive outlook bring out the best in everyone.

When you brainstorm a list of the attributes of a good leader, you begin to realize that complexity and balance are involved. It all depends on the context. Below are some examples of the competing demands you will experience each and every day. We challenge you to add, delete and create a list of your own.

As a charge nurse, you must be:

- a patient's advocate, a physician's partner *and* a peer resource.
- firm and business-like *and* warm and friendly.
- approachable, available *and* completing your own work.
- empathetic *and* emphatic.
- deliberately calm *and* acting quickly in emergencies.
- objective *and* subjective.
- fair *and* arbitrary.
- engaging the team work *and* knocking out tasks.
- managing by fact *and* managing by intuition.
- communicating often *and* thinking always.

14

- making professional decisions *and* making unpopular decisions.
- working the plan *and* open to changing priorities.
- serious *and* light-hearted.
- respectful *and* demanding.

As you can see, leading others is a balancing act. A leader needs to be rigid, flexible, inspiring, demanding, and the list goes on. The trick is using the right approach at the right time. In many ways this reality is similar to patient care. Great clinicians use their knowledge and expertise to size up the situation, choose an appropriate response, and then they intervene with skill. We need our leaders to do the same.

"Leaders stand up for their beliefs and practice what they preach. They show others by their own example that they live by the values they profess. Leaders know that while their position gives them authority, their behavior earns them respect. It is consistency between words and actions that builds a leader's respect." — *Kouzes and Posner, leadership authors*

Personal Lessons

Reflections

- Who are the positive informal leaders on your unit?
  - How did they gain their power? Knowledge? Experience? Kindness? Consistency? Authority? Trustworthiness? Dependability? Fairness?
- What do you need to do to gain the respect of your peers?
  - Which of your behaviors need to change to meet this goal?
  - Who can help you make these changes?
- What do you need to do to meet the expectations of your supervisor?
- If you could develop your skills and abilities in one core area, what would it be?

- How have other charge nurses gained respect on this unit?
- What should I do/not do to be among those ranks?
- What hurdles will I face along the way?
- What five behaviors do I need to exhibit in this role?
- Would you be willing to provide me with feedback along the way?
- Who on this unit can I learn from about these issues? Who is doing it right?

Things to Remember

- If you can master the skill of leading where you have no formal authority over those with whom you are working, research would show that you are well on your way to becoming an effective leader (Avolio, 1999). Individuals with the ability to influence others without the use of formal power have a great skill.
- The combination of skills needed to influence others varies from person to person. Think of someone in your life who has a great deal of power and influence. At times, this comes from their knowledge, extroversion, force, ability to model the way, humor, strong moral compass or work ethic. Any combination of these will serve an individual well. Remember the Five Ps and practice developing and reflecting upon each.
- Remember that reflection and self-awareness are crucial for individual development and growth. If you are not honest with yourself about areas that need to improve, you will stay where you are. Clinical nurses who want to improve their skills must be clear about their deficiencies and consciously work to improve. Developing leadership skills is no different. It is difficult to take a hard look at yourself and admit the need to change, but if you do, you will become stronger and better in your role as charge nurse.

Resources & References

Terms & Acronyms

- **Accountability**—The act of holding someone or oneself responsible to a set of behaviors or standards.
- **Formal Power**—An appointed position or formal authority, similar to that of your boss. Power and authority come with the position. However, much of your job is getting work done through influence (leading).
- **Influence**—*The American Heritage Dictionary* defines influence as "a power affecting a person, thing, or course of events, especially one that operates without any direct or apparent effort." You will need to use influence to remove barriers to improve the efficiency of the systems in your place of work.
- **Informal Power**—Power gained without need of a formal title or position. For instance, think of the person on your unit who everyone looks to even when they are not in charge. This kind of power can be either positive or negative.
- **Self-actualization**—to develop or achieve one's full potential.

Additional Resources

- *Leadership and the One Minute Manager: Increasing Effectiveness Through Situational Leadership* by Ken Blanchard & Patricia Zigarmi
- *Good to Great* by Jim Collins
- *The Leadership Challenge* by Jim Kouzes and Barry Posner
- *Leadership on the Line: Staying Alive through the Dangers of Leading* by Ronald A. Heifetz and Martin Linsky

17

References

Avolio, B. (1999). *Full Leadership Development.* Thousand Oaks, CA: Sage.

Greenleaf, R. (1977). *Servant Leadership*: *A Journey into the Nature of Legitimate Power and Greatness.* New York: Paulist Press.

Chapter Three
A Leader's Resources and Stakeholders

Great leaders know they cannot do it alone. They have the ability and responsibility to engage others in the process. A number of resources are available to help you increase your effectiveness and efficiency in the role of charge nurse and many formal and informal learning opportunities exist to broaden your horizons as you seek to develop yourself both personally and professionally. We assert that effective leaders are people who are adept at reaching out for the appropriate resources. We also assert that a leader is a person who is interested in lifelong learning.

In this chapter we discuss some of the resources available to nurse leaders and touch on some that are internal to your organization. Developmental opportunities, key individuals and departmental resources exist within your organization that will help you grow in your role. We also mention resources external to your organization that may be of interest to you. Likewise we cover some external review and recognition organizations and agencies that provide frameworks and requirements for benchmark healthcare organizations.

Another way to think of the people and organizations that provide you with resources is that they are, in one way or another, stakeholders. They have a vested interest or concern in your actions and performance. They may be personally affected by the way you carry out your role. This would be true of patients, significant others and co-workers. Or the outcome or final product of your work may have an impact on the bigger picture, for example, the goals of the hospital or the relevance of professional and academic organizations. They have a stake in your performance. If you are successful so are they.

This chapter is designed to answer your questions, broaden your horizons, deepen your knowledge, develop your professional interests and advance your career. The more you know about the people and opportunities around you, the more confident you will be in knowing that you have the resources available to succeed as a leader.

"Most people have no idea of the giant capacity we can immediately command when we focus all of our resources on mastering a single area of our lives." — *Tony Robbins, leadership author*

A Key to Success

If you are to be efficient and effective as a charge nurse, you must be comfortable and adept at using the information and communication systems in your facility. We have moved past the age of each person *possessing* a body of knowledge to the age of each person *accessing* knowledge and information. It is no longer necessary to know and remember everything. However, it is necessary to know how to access information and how to navigate information systems. *Become an expert in these systems.*

It is essential for you to be knowledgeable and skilled in the use of the communication links internal and external to your workplace. Know how to alert emergency code team members. Be familiar with the ways to reach key people and departments. Many physicians see patients in several locations and may use various communication devices and systems.

There are many unsung heroes in the Departments of Health Information Technology and Telecommunications—use them. Get to know them.

"The greatest genius will never be worth much if he pretends to draw exclusively from his own resources."—*Johann Wolfgang von Goethe, author, scientist, politician*

Organizational Resources and Stakeholders

Key Individuals and Departments

Patients—They are the reason for our work. Even in the charge nurse position, one step removed from the bedside, the patient's needs are paramount in your actions.

Families and Significant Others—Having a good relationship with family/significant others is like having more staff. Remember what it is like to have someone you care about trying to navigate the healthcare system, and follow the Golden Rule. The trick is to comply with the Health Insurance Portability and Accountability Act (HIPAA) guidelines, yet to be as informative as possible. As charge nurse, you may find it is your role to facilitate communication between significant others and physicians.

Nursing Team—These men and women carry out the plan of action for the day. Team members expect clear direction, a manageable assignment and a positive environment in which to do their work.

Physicians—These professional colleagues are your partners in care. Get to know their personal preferences and work with your team to meet their needs. Not every doctor, even within the same specialty, wants everything done the same way. Know who wants to be called at home in the middle of the night. Know who wants you to call the house staff and know who wants their patients on the teaching service. Know who wants to use intensivists or hospitalists. Know who covers for them when they are having a day off or a vacation. Know who has privileges to do invasive procedures on the unit and know why each doctor is seeing each patient—attending, specialist, consultant, and so forth. Facilitate communication and the passing of vital information among them.

Advanced Practice Nurses (APNs) and Physician Assistants (PAs)—These men and women are experts in specialized areas of patient care. They are valuable resources to you and the physicians with whom you work. APNs are helpful in developing nursing plans of care for unusual or difficult patients.

Student Nurses—Here is where idealism meets reality and the next generation of nurses originates. Be good to these men and women. They need you and you need them. Remember what it was like when you were a student? *Be the nurse you always wanted to be, and they will become that nurse, too.*

Vascular Access Nurse—Know who on your unit is an expert with difficult intravenous starts. Know what resources are available if you need help beyond the members of your team. Consider patient safety and comfort as well as efficiency.

Codes and Code Teams—The appropriate use of emergency codes and knowing the indicators that warrant alerting code teams is sometimes within the role of the charge nurse. Therefore, it is important for you to know when to use and how to summon these resources. Examples are Code Blue Team (CBT), Rapid Response Team (RRT) and High Acuity Response Team (HART). Be knowledgeable, too, of safety codes; for example, Code Pink for child abduction and Code Red for fire.

Support Departments and Staff—Many men and women in the organization provide the expertise, equipment and environment for therapeutic patient care. Patient safety and staff satisfaction are both improved if you have an appreciative relationship with members of support staff. Say hello when one of them is on your unit. Be alert to unfamiliar personnel. Introduce yourself and inquire as to their role in patient care. Take a moment to express your appreciation to these team members. Develop, too, a friendly and appreciative relationship with members of the healthcare team who may never appear on the unit, for example, the finance team.

Expressing appreciation for the work of everyone and developing personal relationships with the "bigger" team improves teamwork. Another important reason for this positive inclusive behavior is that it is one way of acting as a role model for others.

Staff Development—In your workplace there is probably an entire department dedicated to helping you learn and develop. In most cases this is called the Staff Development Department. Take advantage of the many *free* educational offerings provided by them. For example, there are in-services on new clinical technology and classes designed to educate you on information system updates. This resource may also help you to keep abreast of changes in internal policies and procedures and external regulatory or state board of nursing requirements.

It is likely that Staff Development designs the orientation and mentoring programs for your staff. These educators can design classes or guidelines to improve teamwork or work flow on your unit. If you identify an educational need, be sure to communicate this to the staff development department. These men and women are there to assist in meeting learning needs.

Professional Certification—Preparation and testing for many nursing certifications may be available at no or minimal cost within your organization. As you know, many types of certification are available. Preparation for all of them will not be available to you within your organization, but, especially if you work in an acute care setting, you will probably have access to classes in Basic Life Support (BLS), Advanced Life Support (ALS), Pediatric Life Support (PALS), Certification for Acute/Critical Care (CCRN), and, possibly, Sexual Assault Nurse Examiner (SANE). Not only are these classes conveniently located for you, but also taking them with your professional colleagues will build teamwork and relationships.

If you are already certified, you may have an opportunity to serve as an instructor. Teaching is one of the best ways to increase your learning and to build relationships.

Standing Committees—Every work place has a plethora of committees. Serving on one of these is an excellent way to become involved and make a difference. Unit-based and hospital-wide groups often exist to review and improve approaches dedicated to patient outcomes, patient safety and patient satisfaction. Volunteer to be a member.

Task Forces and Work Groups—Prior to the implementation of new work systems and information upgrades there may be an opportunity for you to participate in groups that are dedicated to this purpose. Task forces may also be formed in preparation for review by external organizations such as Joint Commission for Accreditation of Healthcare Organizations (JCAHO), Magnet Recognition or Malcolm Baldrige Review. These groups usually have a shorter time commitment than standing committees. Involvement will provide you with the opportunity to have input, to educate you on the reason for the changes and to prepare you to be a change agent.

Employee Councils—Some healthcare organizations have councils designed for administrators and front-line employees to share information. These cabinets are excellent forums for you to get a glimpse of the "bigger" picture and to have the opportunity to share what it is like "in the trenches." Your supervisor will know if a council of this nature exists in your organization and can assist you in becoming a member.

Your Supervisor—This person's role is to provide you with education, guidance, counseling and feedback. S/He is there to answer your questions and to assist you in doing your job. Your supervisor can provide you with information on what is expected and how your work will be evaluated. Remember that people usually like to be asked for advice and guidance. Your supervisor has a unique perspective. Discussing your future will be helpful to you and will impress upon your supervisor that you are serious about your career. If you wish to be a member of a committee or task force, this is the person who can be your sponsor.

Nursing Administration and Other Administrators—Make sure you are aware of who these men and women are. Introduce yourself when you have the opportunity. You will find it interesting to know about their role in delivering health care. They, in turn, will be interested in getting to know you. You may serve with them on committees and they may become future mentors.

Mentor—The role of mentor is to help you as you learn and develop. The great thing about mentoring is that both parties benefit. Relationships with mentors sometimes last a lifetime. Remember, you can have multiple mentors and they do not all need to be formal relationships. Consider, too, becoming a mentor for others.

External Resources and Stakeholders

Developmental Opportunities

Beyond the walls of your organization are many resources designed to expand your growth and development.

Continuing Education Units (CEUs)—Many states require nurses to earn continuing education units for renewal of licenses. It is true, also, that most nurses are interested in professional lifelong learning. For this reason the market place has responded with many ways to earn CEUs.

Enter "nursing CEUs" into your search engine and many sites dedicated to this purpose will pop up. Taking CEUs online is often a quick and convenient way to fulfill licensure requirements. If you prefer self-study or find it inconvenient to attend group classes this approach may work for you. Always verify that the CEUs have been accredited by your state board of nursing or by the American Nurse Credentialing Center (ANCC). Unaccredited units will probably not be accepted to fulfill licensure renewal requirements.

Many vendors provide CEU group classes in the community setting. You probably receive notification of some of these via email or "snail" mail. Learning in a group setting can be a vehicle for you to become acquainted with other nurses in your geographical area. These classes are usually large and do not lend themselves to asking questions nor to group discussion. Again, check to make sure that the vendor offers accredited CEUs.

Nearby colleges and universities that grant nursing degrees usually provide continuing education classes. Attending these classes, which are often available in the evening, is an excellent way to further your professional knowledge and to earn CEUs. University-based continuing education classes are usually small and taught by nursing professionals from the surrounding community. There is opportunity for group discussion, Q & A, and networking.

Professional publications, journals and books are other developmental resources. These sources are available to you online, at university libraries and by joining professional organizations.

Pursuing Certification and Advanced Degree—You may be interested in becoming certified in a specialized area of nursing. The website for American Nurses Credentialing Center (ANCC) is www.nursecredentialing.org. Here you will find all the information you need to pursue certification in specialty practice areas. Information is easily available about the many different types of certification, the requirements to earn this recognition, and the location of testing site.

One of the best ways to advance your career and professional development is to earn an advanced degree. Universities and colleges near you may offer this opportunity. Many schools offer evening and part-time programs and it is also possible for you to earn advanced academic credits and degrees online.

Here are a just few of the many websites that may help you.

- *American Association of Colleges of Nursing* (www.aacn.nche.edu) has listings of colleges and universities with nursing programs and sources of financial aid.
- *Nursing Link* (nursinglink.monster.com) lists career and educational resources as well as job opportunities.

- *Lippincott's Nursing Center* (www.nursingcenter.org) has similar content as well as information about certified and advanced nursing practice.
- *Nurse Zone* (www.nursezone.com) offers information about financial aid and creating resumes.
- *Accredited Online Schools and Colleges* (www.accreditedonlincolleges.org) lists degree-granting colleges and universities in the United States.
- *Discover Nursing* (www.discovernursing.com) has information about various nursing career options.

Your supervisor can help you coordinate your work and class schedules. Also, check with your human resources department to find out if earning certification or an advanced degree qualifies you for a better pay grade or makes you eligible for career advancement. Organizations seeking Magnet Recognition may require nurses to seek advanced degrees, and therefore, reward that achievement with salary increases.

State Board of Nursing—The website for your state board of nursing is a valuable resource to learn about the laws applicable to nursing in the state where you practice. Enter into your search engine the name of your state followed by "Board of Nursing" to access the website. You will find the rules and regulations that govern your practice, as well as position papers on various aspects of nursing, licensure, CEU requirements and much more.

Volunteering—Offering your services as a professional volunteer is a great way to build your self-confidence and to increase your awareness of the community around you. There may be opportunities at senior centers or in the schools or churches that serve your area. State and local government committees may welcome the input of a registered nurse in the process of creating policies that have some bearing on the health and welfare of citizens. Explore the opportunities around you. You will not only be giving back to the community, but also developing yourself. A word of caution: check to be sure your malpractice insurance covers you as a volunteer.

Review and Regulatory Organizations—There are organizations whose purpose and mission it is to review, regulate and recognize healthcare organizations. Following are a few of these agencies. One of the resources available to you is online access to the wealth of information that these organizations have amassed. Standards of patient care, examples of benchmark performance organizations and models of care delivery are a few of the helpful ideas you will find.

- Joint Commission on Accreditation of Healthcare Organizations (JCAHO)—JCAHO is an independent organization that reviews and recognizes healthcare organizations. Criteria for review can be seen at the JCAHO website, www.jointcommission.org.
- State Boards of Health—the board of health in your state may license mother/baby care centers. Information about the state requirements is available to you online. In most states the board of health is required to follow up on any citizen concerns or complaints about care. Online access is available to state healthcare rules and laws.
- Magnet Recognition Program—The American Credentialing Center, a subsidiary of the American Nurses Association, surveys, appraises and recognizes nursing services that seek Magnet Designation. The Magnet Program promotes safe, positive work environments. Information about successful approaches is available online at www.nursecredentialing.org.
- The Malcolm Baldrige National Quality Award recognizes organizations of all types for performance excellence. It is administered by the National Institute of Standards and Technology. Comprehensive criteria specific for healthcare organizations are available at www.nist.gov/baldrige.
- Sigma Theta Tau International (STTI) is an honorary nursing society that recognizes individual student nurses and nurse leaders for academic and clinical excellence. Criteria for membership and a wealth of information can be found at www.nursingsociety.org.

Professional Organizations—Joining a professional nursing organization is a great ways to learn and to stay current in your field or specialty. As an organizational member you are eligible to receive professional journals and attend annual conferences. Both of these venues offer CEUs and educational activities. Professional organizations may offer certification classes, career assistance and access to website information that may not be available to nonmembers.

Professional organizations exist at the national, state and local levels. Attendance at meetings and conventions provides the opportunity to meet nurses with similar interests. Presentation of papers and publication of articles is also possible through this avenue.

You will find that nearly every nursing specialty and many special interest groups have professional organizations. Following is a list of a few of the nursing societies that may interest you.
- American Nursing Association (ANA)— www.nursingworld.org.
- American Organization of Nurse Executives (AONE)— www.aone.org.
- Academy of Medical-Surgical Nurses (AMSN) — www.amsn.org.
- American Association of Critical-Care Nurses (AACN)— www.aacn.org.
- Emergency Nurses Association (ENA)— www.ena.org.
- Association of Women's Health, Obstetrical and Neonatal Nurses (AWHONN)— awhonn.org.
- American Association of periOperative Registered Nurses (AORN)— aorn.org.
- American Psychiatric Nurses Association (APNA)— www.apna.org.
- American Association of Ambulatory Care Nursing (AAACN)— www.aaacn.org.

In addition to the publications from professional organizations there are many excellent nursing journals and magazines. Here are a few.

- American Journal of Nursing (AJN)—journals.lww.com/ajnonline.
- Nursing Management—journals.lww.com/nursingmanagement
- Journal of Nursing Administration (JONA)—journals.lww.com/jonanournal.
- Evidence-Based Practice (EBP) Network—www.nursingcenter.com/evidencebasedpracticenetwork.

"Happiness, to me, lies in stretching, to the farthest boundaries of which we are capable, the resources of the mind and heart."
— *Leo Calvin Rosten, author and political philosopher*

Conclusion

While the magnitude of this information may feel a bit overwhelming, rest assured that there are people, departments, and organizations with a vested interest in your success. So rather than feel like you need to investigate all of these at once, simply pick one or two that may meet your needs at this time. Then, revisit this guidebook periodically and you will be amazed at how much you are learning as a leader.

Personal Lessons

Reflections

- Place a checkmark by the resources in this chapter that you already use. Where are your strengths and opportunities?
- Circle the resources that you consider to be future opportunities.
- What educational resources are offered by your organization to improve your knowledge, skills and abilities as a leader?
- What are the committees at your institution that interest you?
- Does your institution reward additional credentials?

- The charge nurse is the person who reaches out for the appropriate resources and brings them to bear on each situation—moment-to-moment and patient-to-patient.
- It is no longer necessary to know and remember everything. *However, it is necessary to know how to access information and how to navigate information systems.*
- Getting involved is exciting and fulfilling. You will meet some wonderful people. Volunteering to teach in-services and classes is the best way to learn. Read as much as you can. Take advantage of the many resources available to nurses.
- Utilize your resources. There is no need to "go it alone." Not only will you be better at your job, you will save time.
- Joining a professional organization or preparing for certification are great ways to help you in your continuing professional development.
- There are many stakeholders who have a vested interest in how well you do your job. If you are successful so are they.

Case Study—Grace

Grace's supervisor recently assigned her to the duty of charge nurse saying, "I have great faith in your technical competence and know you will be great in the role." This makes Grace feel good considering she has only been a nurse for one year. Grace is all business when it comes to getting her work done. She does not spend much time gossiping or chumming around with the other nurses. To her, the patient comes first. She spends little time getting to know her teammates and doesn't bother going to the charge nurse in-services. It is no surprise to others on her unit when she is assigned to charge, but some are worried that she will try to rule with an "iron fist" and expect everyone else around her to work the same way she does. Mark, a nurse of 23 years, even goes so far as to say that he will not follow Grace's lead. She is young, naïve and insensitive to the needs of her teammates in Mark's eyes. Others agree.

Grace is unaware of these feelings. Her supervisor (Jill) is aware, but thinks the charge nurse experience will be good for Grace's development. She plans to wait and see how things unfold in the first couple of weeks. Besides, Jill does not have the time to hold Grace's hands, as JCAHO is due for a visit. She has to spend a lot of time in meetings and at the computer. Jill figures that unless she gets a lot of complaints from physicians everything is okay.

Review Questions:

- What are the red flags in this story?
- How will Grace effectively lead those around her?
- What are the barriers that Grace will face?
- What resources are available to Grace?
- What can Jill do to help Grace become a better leader?

Case Study—Penny

Penny has been a charge nurse for 10 years. She loves being in charge and likes everyone with whom she works. She bends over backwards to cover for others and ensures that everything runs smoothly on her watch. As a result, everything seems to be running like clockwork. She loves the fact that everyone feels comfortable coming to her with problems and she loves being part of the solution, even if it means that she needs to move into a frontline role from time to time to get things back on track.

Lately, Penny's supervisor has been on her case because she noticed that Penny is not holding co-workers accountable. To Penny, these issues are minimal and she blows them off as "one time" events. Penny likes being the hero. She fixes errors and finishes incomplete assignments. Doctors are always telling her she is the best and they would be "lost" without her.

Pressure from her supervisor to slow down and confront inappropriate behavior has been mounting. Penny thinks it will pass. Her boss is determined to coach her to delegate and to hold others accountable.

Review Questions:

- What are the red flags in this story?
- How does Penny need to change? What are some reasons she is resisting?
- What are the barriers that Penny faces if she changes?
- What resources are available to Penny?

Resources & References

Terms & Acronyms

- **Accreditation**—The process by which an organization or an institution is recognized for meeting predetermined standards. Also the process by which an organization determines that course content meets minimum requirements. Examples of organizations that grant accreditation are the Joint Commission on Accreditation of Health Care Organizations (JCAHO) and the American Nurse Credentialing Center (ANCC).
- **Benchmark performance**—Measurement of outcomes compared to others in the field or against specific criteria.
- **Certification**—The act of authorizing legality or legitimacy or of granting credit or recognition.
- **Change Agent**—Someone who knows and understands the dynamics that facilitate or hinder change. Someone who acts to alter human capability or organizational systems to a higher degree of output or self-actualization.
- **Hospitalist**—A dedicated in-patient physician who works exclusively in a hospital and may assume the medical care for a primary care physician during a patient's hospitalization.
- **Intensivist**—A board-certified physician who is additionally certified in the subspecialty of critical care medicine.
- **Models of care**—Frameworks for delivering nursing care and education to patients/clients.

- **Policies and Procedures**—Written documents that detail the clinical, business, and other practices of the organization.
- **Stakeholder**—a person or organization with an interest or concern in your performance or whose own success can be affected by your actions.

Additional Resources

- *Achieving Success Through Social Capital: Tapping Hidden Resources in Your Personal and Business Networks* by Wayne E. Baker

Chapter Four
Self-Awareness

"Know thyself." — *Socrates, Greek philosopher, 470-399 BC*

Your ability to lead and influence others will be maximized if you are more fully self-aware. We briefly touch on this notion in the previous chapter but it is a concept that deserves special attention.

The challenge of self-awareness is the sheer number of dimensions in which you have to grasp your strengths and weaknesses. For instance, when it comes to leadership you need to be aware of your approach to conflict, communication style, responses to stress, emotional intelligence, social intelligence, locus of control, motivation to lead, self-efficacy, attention to detail, influence strategies, and so on. This list can seem a bit overwhelming *and* daunting or it may be energizing and exciting. The good news is that you already have a strong grasp on many of the above-mentioned attributes—there are likely only three or four that need some deliberate practice.

Here is a hard truth. Even if you do not have a strong grasp or awareness in each of the above-mentioned realms, *others do.* Those with whom you work experience your great strengths and areas for development each and every day. They live them. Just as you live with theirs. So it is critical that you have allies who are willing to provide you with unfiltered and unsolicited feedback. If you can build these relationships with pragmatic, no-nonsense, individuals you will have direct access to crucial feedback.

You may hear things like, "you tend to avoid conflict," "your attitude can bring others down at times," or "some feel that you do not work as hard as you could." This feedback is worth its weight in gold because you now know where to tweak your behavior.

So self-awareness can be boiled down to a very simple notion. Do you have a strong grasp on your strengths and weaknesses in multiple domains? Do your perceptions of self align with the perceptions of others who know you best? If there is a strong alignment, then you are self-aware. However, if you have an inflated or a deflated sense of self, then further exploration is needed. Think about the men and women you work with—who of your peers has a balanced and healthy sense of self? Who is a little over confident in their worth or who undervalues their contributions to the team? Great leaders are self-aware.

"I think self-awareness is probably the most important thing towards being a champion." — *Billie Jean King, tennis pro*

Other Levels of Awareness

Another level of awareness requires discussion. As you know, registered nurses are thrust into a societal role that puts them at great risk for poor self-esteem and ineffective performance if they are not self-aware. Many reasons exist for this, and they can be placed into three general categories.

1. The nursing profession attracts people who want to help others. This is good; however, there is a pathological or adverse side to wanting to help others. It is called being an enabler. The personality traits of an enabler include being over-responsible, placatory, self-critical, and victimized and they may unconsciously worsen the problems of others. Some nurses are enablers and have issues with self-esteem. Communication coming from enablers is not always straightforward which further complicates an already complex environment.
2. Although society recognizes nurses as professionals, they do not have all of the benefits (or risks) that society would generally recognize as being in the domain of a professional. Nurses actually function somewhere between a "blue-collar" and a "white-collar" world, which can cause conflict. Sometimes nurses *act* as professionals and sometimes they do not. This is often

dictated by the circumstance in which they find themselves. Moreover, sometimes nurses are *treated* as professionals, and sometimes they are not. For example, in our society, professionals are usually not paid by the hour and they are not required to request permission to work overtime to complete the work they may be doing for a client. On the other hand, they are expected to complete the work at hand without additional pay.

3. Nurses work in a stressful, exacting, demanding, highly charged environment. A nurse's work is not done in isolation and requires intense interaction with many people. It is inevitable that there will be conflicting priorities, verbal demands, strong emotions, ethical dilemmas, competing commitments and criticism.

These dynamics exist in any healthcare organization so it's helpful to be aware of them and to learn ways to navigate through these subtle complexities. It's important to know that some of these realities "eat people up inside" even though they may not be aware that it is happening. For example, think of a colleague who is unhappy in the role of nurse but cannot quite put his finger on why. It could be he is struggling with #2 above.

Self-awareness will help you cope and even thrive in a complex environment. You cannot control the way that people speak and act toward you, but you *can* control the way *you* speak and act. Appropriate messages and actions on your part will have a profound effect on taking the emotion out of a situation and make communication more calm and professional. Best of all, the *patient* will remain the focus instead of the conflict among caregivers. *This is a charge nurse's goal — to keep the focus on the patient at all times.*

So as your never-ending journey toward a more enlightened and self-aware existence continues, we would like to bring your attention to two final concepts: managing triggers and accepting criticism.

"**Explore thyself. Herein are demanded the eye and the nerve.**"—*Henry David Thoreau, author, poet, philosopher*

Triggers and Buttons

In 1967, Thomas Harris wrote a book entitled *I'm OK-You're OK*. It discusses our relationships and interactions in terms of how we view ourselves. He describes three basic scenarios: *I'm not OK-You're OK*, *I'm OK-You're not OK*, and *I'm OK-You're OK*. The concept is easy to understand and very helpful in learning about oneself.

The concept makes you really think about what internal triggers cause you to react and respond in the way you do. The environment in which charge nurses work is fraught with triggers. Thinking through what makes you communicate in an ineffective or destructive manner is essential if you are to be an effective charge nurse. Then you can identify and control these triggers and *choose* your response—to act rather than react.

A classic work that expands on the topic of self-awareness as it relates to leadership is the book *Primal Leadership* by Daniel Goleman, Richard Boyatzis and Annie McKee.

An experience "triggered" me (Cathy) when I was very new in the role of charge nurse that illustrates our point. I approached a physician when he was on the unit to see a particular patient. I stated that the nurse providing direct care to the patient had asked if the doctor could write a certain order. The physician put his face close to mine and said in a very loud voice, "Do I look like an *attending* to you? I am a consultant!" Fortunately, he turned on his heel and walked off the unit. His message and style was a trigger that could have caused me to react unprofessionally. Fortunately there was no time for me to respond. In this case, I found humor in his answer to my question. However, laughing would have been as destructive as spouting off, which might have been another reaction.

Many people who write about leadership talk about *taking your time* before responding to any communication that evokes an emotional reaction in you. Slow down, take a deep breath and think about what you are about to say. A few seconds of reflection are usually all you need to become aware of your feelings. Then you are much more likely to appropriately manage your emotions and respond in a constructive way. Between stimulus and response, you have the ability to *choose your response*. Doing so moves you from the position of victim to one of self-determination. Likewise, beginning your response with "I" or "The patient" usually brings forth a more assertive (rather than passive or aggressive) statement than beginning your response with "You."

Criticism—Is it a Gift?

Perhaps the single best moment to actively practice self-awareness, self-management and the management of triggers is while receiving criticism (or it's more gentle cousin "feedback"). Criticism is something all of us must learn to accept. As a charge nurse, you will have ample opportunities to reflect on reactions to criticism. Why? Everyone in a leadership role receives criticism (e.g., your supervisor, the CEO, the patient's family). At times it's deserved and other times it's a little unfair. As we discussed, one of the steps toward becoming self-aware is in understanding how others perceive you. Sometimes you do not present yourself as you think you do. It is helpful to know this. Being known as a person who is open to feedback and learning how to accept criticism is one way to obtain this information.

People find it difficult to give constructive feedback to one another. Doing so effectively is both skill and art. Often, the messenger is anxious, and their delivery may be hurtful or abrupt. Know and remember this truth. If you can filter the facts and helpful hints from the delivery style, criticism can be managed more successfully. Perhaps more important, incorporate what you have learned into your leadership style and learn how to provide others with feedback in a positive and constructive manner.

So is criticism a gift? We are not sure. Perhaps it is more like a white elephant gift. Awkwardly packaged, a bit off the mark but it just may be an unexpected treasure.

"The one important thing I have learned over the years is the difference between taking one's work seriously and taking one's self seriously. The first is imperative and the second is disastrous." — *Dame Margot Fonteyn, British ballerina*

A Never-Ending Process

Years ago, an elderly patient gave me some feedback that helped me become more self-aware. That evening, I (Cathy) felt there was too much to do and not enough time. Most inconveniently, a patient put on his call light. When I went to his room my non-verbal behavior must have been screaming, "I don't have time for this." He took one look at me and said, "Never mind, I'll save my question for someone else. I can see you are in too much of a rush to be a good nurse." Ouch! This incident occurred more than 20 years ago, but I will never forget his words. They stung. They were pointed. They were hard to swallow. He was right.

Like learning to lead, self-awareness is a process that is never completed. Develop the habit of reflecting upon the events of the day and think about how you reacted and why. This practice is called self-monitoring or meta-cognition and some scholars feel it is one of the most important tools for any leader. Others call it critical reflection, which some psychologists suggest is a core tenant of how adults develop and grow. Perhaps most important, self-awareness leads to alignment of verbal and non-verbal behavior and quiets the struggle between your internal voice and your external life.

"The outward freedom that we shall attain will only be in exact proportion to the inward freedom to which we may have grown at a given moment. And if this is a correct view of freedom, our chief energy must be concentrated on achieving reform from within."—*Gandhi, Indian leader*

Personal Lessons

A Quick Self-Awareness Assessment

Rank yourself using a scale from 1-7 in which "1" is *strongly disagree* and "7" is *strongly agree*, on the following questions.

- I manage my emotions well with co-workers.
- My perception of myself aligns well with the perceptions that others have of me.
- I have a strong interest in becoming more self-aware.
- Critical reflection is a habit or way of being for me.
- I regulate my emotions when my "buttons" are being pushed.
- I am known as someone who is open to feedback.
- I know when my mood negatively affects the moods of others around me.
- I have the communication skills to work through most situations.
- I am a self-aware individual.

How did you score? If you scored three or less on an item, it may be an area for improvement. Think about it.

Reflections

- What "triggers" take you over the edge when working with physicians, other departments, your peers and so forth?
- What happens when you "go over the edge"? Do you withdraw? Yell? Communicate through the issues? Gossip? Talk to everyone *but* the person you need to?
- What do you do to manage your emotions in heated discussions?
- How well do you control your emotions? Can others (e.g., patients, families, peers) quickly see your mood? How do they respond?
- Do you have a trusted confidant who is willing to provide you with unfiltered and unbiased feedback?

41

- Have you seen peers "derail" on the job? What did this behavior look like and what caused it? Was there anything you could have done to help the person regain self-control?

Things to Remember

- Your mood is contagious and influences those around you. Generally speaking, if your moods are positive and upbeat, that is good. However, toxic attitudes and behaviors are destructive to you and those with whom you work.
- Leaders who have a good system for recognizing their emotions and at the same time regulating them will likely go far in an organization.
- Individuals who are open to feedback from others will likely have a better interpretation of how others perceive them. Moreover, they are better equipped to adjust their behavior.

Case Study—Rosalee

Rosalee has been a nurse for more than 10 years. She knows everything there is to know about the unit and knows all of the doctors and managers. Rosalee has excellent clinical skills. Doctors and nurses respect her for this expertise.

However, when she is in charge she acts like a dictator. She is a "know-it-all" and can be condescending to those with whom she works. In her effort to run a "tight ship" she barks orders and is overly critical of the team. Rosalee seems unaware that she is disliked as a leader. No one knows how to confront her. People are afraid that if they say something to Rosalee, they will get in trouble with the nurse manager with whom she is close.

Review Questions:

- Do you think Rosalee is aware of how her behavior affects her co-workers?
- How will Rosalee do as a leader?

- What could those around her do to help Rosalee become more self-aware?
- If team members choose to do nothing, how are they a part of the dysfunctional environment?
- What could Rosalee do to improve teamwork so that the focus remains on the patient(s) instead of her behavior?

Resources & References

Terms & Acronyms

- **Criticism**—Criticism is evaluation, assessment, appraisal analysis or judgment of some aspect of your work or your person. It may be positive or negative. Learn to appreciate criticism (and feedback) as an opportunity for reflection and growth. If you are known as a person who is open to feedback, you will have more input and a better understanding of how you can improve and how people perceive you.
- **Self-Awareness**—An awareness of your own strengths and areas of growth.
- **Self-Determination**—State of being able to manage yourself independent of the influence or control of another.
- **Self-Management**—The regulation of emotions so that your response is appropriate for a given situation.
- **Triggers & Buttons**—Events or situations that cause, evoke or set off responses in you.

Additional Resources

- *Hard Won Wisdom*: *More Than 50 Extraordinary Women Mentor You to Find Self-Awareness, Perspective, and Balance* by Fawn Germer
- *Don't Give It Away*: *A Workbook of Self-Awareness and Self-Affirmations for Young Women* by Iyanla Vanzant
- *Visualization — an Introductory Guide*: *Use Visualization to Improve Your Health and Develop Your Self-awareness and Creativity* by Helen Graham

- *Primal leadership*: *Realizing the power of emotional intelligence* by Daniel Goleman, Richard Boyatzis, & Annie McKee
- *Crucial Conversations: Tools for Talking When Stakes Are High* by Kerry Patterson, Joseph Grenny, Ron McMillan, and Al Switzler

References

Harris, T. (1967). *I'm OK-You're OK*. New York: Harper & Row, Publishers, Inc.

Chapter Five
Patient Safety & Error Prevention

"Nursing is above all a provocative calling. Year by year, nurses have to learn new and improved methods. Year by year, nurses are called upon to do more and better than they have ever done." — *Florence Nightengale*

It is startling to realize that patient safety and error prevention did not become of prime importance to healthcare organizations until the very end the 20th century. Prior to that time these concepts were existent but of much less importance in strategic plans and quality initiatives. In 1999 the Institute of Medicine (IOM) published a report entitled *To Err is Human: Building a Safer Health System which* suggested that between 44,000 and 98,000 people in the United States die annually because of errors in patient care. This report caught the attention of the media, the public, third party payers and healthcare providers. It was much quoted and discussed and led to further studies and reports. The most important result from these reports and studies is that it inspired the healthcare industry to look more objectively at its practices and outcomes. It caused us to make changes in the way health care is provided and the quality indicators we monitor. It changed how we lead.

My initial response to the IOM study was denial and disbelief. Upon reflection I (Cathy) began to realize that within healthcare organizations there is a sort of "conspiracy of silence" about errors and "near misses" that happen or almost happen to patients. I thought back to a scene that took place when I was a student nurse. In my initial surgical rotation I scrubbed in on a case as an observer. During intubation the patient's front tooth was dislodged. A voice at the table said, "No one saw this happen." I was shocked. It was the first time I had witnessed the harming of a patient. It was an accident and, of course, not intentional. But the fact that a "cover-up" was the first verbalized plan to handle this harm to a patient was unconscionable to me. I discussed the event with my nursing instructor. She assured me it was only a casual remark, maybe even an attempt at humor. But I thought about the words a lot and have never forgotten that moment. Nor have I forgotten the way I felt about it.

Unfortunately, almost every nurse has had an encounter with the wrong side of patient safety. We have found errors made by others, experienced a "near miss" or even made an error ourselves. Chances are that if you have made an error you will never forget it. Making a mistake leaves a lasting memory of how easily it can happen. It makes you a believer in reform. Any change in process or procedure that will prevent errors and harm to patients is definitely a good idea.

Many errors do not result in adverse outcomes. They may not even be discovered or reported. It has been difficult to replicate the 1999 findings of IOM because there is not a standard approach to defining, recording and reporting errors. Many questions have arisen. What is the definition of a medical error? How are medical errors counted? Is a "near-miss" counted as an error, that is, if an error is caught and corrected before the patient is touched? Are errors that result in no adverse outcome counted? How are errors reported? To whom are they reported? In spite of these questions it is our role to prevent errors and to keep patients safe.

Errors happen and patient safety is vulnerable because our systems and processes are not as error-proof as they should and can be. It is inherent in the nature of healthcare professionals to feel personally responsible and accountable for patient safety. However, it is often the fault of complex and imperfect processes that errors occur. Delivery care systems are, therefore, the focus of scrutiny and reform. Can we make our processes simpler, more foolproof and secure? How can we change systems and equipment to prevent errors in the future? These are the questions we must constantly ask ourselves. Studying errors with the process known as root-cause analysis helps to uncover system breakdowns.

Continuous improvement does not result from thinking in terms of who is at fault or who is to blame for an error. Continuous improvement comes from studying every error and "near miss" to better understand how the *process or system* can be changed to prevent or decrease the likelihood of errors in the future.

Continuous improvement will happen more quickly if people feel that reporting an error is an expected practice. Reporting will lead to greater safety for patients. A lack of reporting is a barrier to safety. There is reticence to come forward when people feel that doing so will get them or another person "in trouble." We are making progress in creating blame-free environments and increasing patient safety, but we have a long way to go. In fact, this journey will never end.

One of the ways we can continuously improve care is to create an environment of acceptance and forgiveness instead of one of blame and fear. When an error is made and reported, it is an opportunity to investigate the root cause(s) and then change the systems or processes that have allowed an unsafe act to occur. The creation of safer systems and processes must happen if we are to reach our goal of zero tolerance for errors.

It is possible that as charge nurse you will have the responsibility for following up when an error has been made. Be proactive, but not punitive. Ask your supervisor for guidance when you are first learning the error reporting and investigation process.

"It may seem strange to enunciate as the very first requirement in a hospital that it should do the sick no harm." — *Florence Nightengale*

Patient Safety is a Priority

You are responsible for leading many tasks as a charge nurse. The most important of these is the safety of the patients. Your top priority is patient safety. You have to help everyone remember safety is his or her priority too. You are the patient's advocate.

Clarity in communication is the best way to meet this challenge. Special care must be taken when receiving verbal orders. Repeating what you have heard is an excellent way to clarify that the sender and receiver agree upon what has been said. Be precise about what you are delegating and what you expect to be done.

Resolving conflicts and calming emotions are important factors in the prevention of errors. Subjective studies have shown an inverse link between disruptive behaviors and patient safety. A review of these studies is available online in the August, 2008 issue of *The Joint Commission Journal of Quality and Patient Safety*. A majority of the doctors and nurses that responded suggested that disruptive behavior causes adverse events and medical errors, and has an adverse effect on patient safety, patient mortality, quality of care and patient satisfaction.

Fortunately, much has happened since the IOM report in 1999. Recommendations that improve patient safety and that are based on scientific evidence in the form of improved patient outcomes are now commonplace. External regulatory agencies and third party payers are all demanding changes. Good suggestions are coming to us from within and outside the healthcare industry and many are being implemented. For instance, the adoption of electronic information systems has helped resolve the issues of illegible handwriting, transcription errors and incompatible orders. *However, it still comes down to the person-to-person interaction that is the essence of health care*. No amount of changes in systems will substitute for each person taking personal responsibility for what they do, or do not do, for the patient.

"The safety of the people is the supreme law." — *Cicero, Roman philosopher, 106-43 BC*

Health Care is Becoming Safer

Some of what must be done is beyond the control of an individual nurse, but it helps to know how intensely health care is being scrutinized and how seriously we must take the issue of patient safety. It also helps to know that we are surrounded by efforts designed to make our practice safer.

Soon after the IOM report, a group of *Fortune 500* executives external to health care formed the Leapfrog Group. The organizations that founded this group were the largest purchasers of healthcare coverage. Their interest stemmed not only from their concern that their employees were receiving safe care, but also from their concern regarding the exorbitant cost of health care. Every error costs money. They wanted to know that good dollars were not being wasted on bad medicine. The Leapfrog Group studied the hospital environment.

As objective observers and consumers, and with the help of experts skilled at designing safe environments, The Leapfrog Group made some suggestions. The three initial recommendations proposed by the Leapfrog Group were:

1. Implementation of Computerized Physician Order Entry (CPOE).
2. Critical care units staffed with physicians trained as intensivists.
3. Evidence-based hospital referral for high-risk procedures. Patients should be directed to healthcare organizations for high-risk surgeries and procedures based upon the number of similar procedures done by that healthcare organization, as well as the history of outcomes. In other words, complex procedures should be done in places where there is evidence that a large number of these procedures have been done safely and with success.

These suggestions make sense. Many healthcare organizations have implemented them. The Leapfrog Group continues to be involved in studying and making recommendations for patient safety. Their website (www.leapfroggroup.org) is rich with findings and data relevant to the topic of patient safety.

A recent Leapfrog Group recommendation is that healthcare organizations use safe practices endorsed by the National Quality Forum (NQF). See www.qualityforum.org. NQF is a nonprofit organization that is dedicated to improving health care through gaining consensus on national performance improvement goals, endorsing standards, public reporting of outcomes, education and outreach. You will find valuable information about their activities and findings at their website.

Many organizations have become leaders in the work of improving health care. The organization you work for probably works with many of them. On your unit, it is likely that you collect data that is indicative of the quality of clinical care. The amount of information available on the topic of patient safety and error prevention is overwhelming. Ideas and initiatives abound. Fortunately, there is evidence that suggests that errors are decreasing. The patient is safer and more error free. However, there is much work yet to do.

Unfortunately, there are still obstacles that impede rapid, wide-scale adaptation of some of the recommended changes. The barriers are expense, the physician reimbursement system, traditional referral patterns and the trend toward every community healthcare organization offering nearly every procedure. Universal implementation of recommended changes will take time and money. Some of these changes reach beyond the ability of individual healthcare organizations to fix. They require changes in the "larger system."

"You wouldn't just decide to forget about recovering the black box after an air crash. So why should it be thought so strange to learn from every accident in health care?" — *Sir Liam Donaldson, British physician and author*

JCAHO and Safety

The Joint Commission for the Accreditation of Healthcare Organizations (JCAHO) has always had patient safety embedded in its criteria. Beginning in 2003, JCAHO implemented *National Patient Safety Goals*, which are specific and excellent objectives. Each year these are updated and expanded. Healthcare organizations are monitored for compliance to these goals, and accreditation hinges upon implementation and compliance. Progress in technology and agreed upon industry standards are reflected as the National Patient Safety Goals are changed and refined. Visit www.jcaho.org for the latest updates. The website abounds with information regarding the current National Patient Safety Goals, and also information on certification, onsite reviews, reporting requirements, standards of care and ongoing quality initiatives.

"The healthcare system, as it is currently structured, cannot consistently deliver effective care in a safe, timely and efficient manner." — *Institute of Medicine*

The Institute for Healthcare Improvement

As a leader in health care you will find it informative and interesting to become familiar with the work of the Institute for Healthcare Improvement (IHI). This is an organization that has been working for many years through multidisciplinary collaboratives to improve the way we deliver care to patients. Visit their website at www.ihi.org. They do exciting and hopeful work through real caregivers working in real healthcare settings. You will find improvement changes that your healthcare organization has implemented, for example, Rapid Response Teams. You may also find other ideas that would be helpful to you and your healthcare team.

Nursing Care and Patient Safety

All who study patient safety generally agree that nurses as individuals, and as a professional group, are amenable to changes that will benefit patients. In fact, evidence suggests that nurses are *more* likely to see the need for and to admit that change is needed than other healthcare professionals. Perhaps this is because nurses are at the bedside and witness errors and the negative consequences to patients.

In any case, the nursing profession has become astute and proactive at monitoring patient outcomes that are the direct result of nursing interventions (or a lack thereof). Nurses identify and define key indicators, monitor patient outcomes and, from the results, create *databases of nursing actions* that have a direct effect on the well-being of patients.

Resources to learn more about quality initiatives in your organization are available from your supervisor and the Performance Improvement Department. If you do not already have access to the results for your unit and for other units in the organization, ask to see them. Results are probably reported periodically in a scorecard format with comparison to past performance, goals and other departments or organizations.

National Database of Nursing Quality Indicators

The American Nurses Association (ANA) has developed the National Database of Quality Indicators (NDNQI) (www.nursingquality.org). The mission of NDNQI is to help registered nurses in patient safety and quality improvement efforts by providing "researched-based national comparative data on nursing care and the relationship to patient outcomes." Participating hospitals submit data on a regular basis and receive unit-level reports with comparisons to like units. Data is emerging that supports the theory that nurse staffing is related to patient outcomes. Although it makes intuitive sense that adequate staffing and sufficient RNs on a unit result in better outcomes for patients the NDNQI work is providing data to support this supposition.

Some indicators collected regarding RNs are nursing staff skill mix, nursing hours per patient day, nurse education/certification, nurse turnover and nursing satisfaction.

Nurse-sensitive clinical indicators are also collected to study the theory that units with an RN rich staff have a lower incidence of poor patient outcomes. Some of these clinical indicators are: patient falls, hospital-acquired pressure ulcers, peripheral intravenous infiltration, catheter associated urinary tract infections, central line associated blood stream infections and ventilator associated pneumonia.

You can see how having access to this comparative data is helpful to nursing administrators and finance staff when nursing budgets are developed. An argument based upon patient safety and error prevention can be made to support the cost of more registered nurses. The benefit and cost of adequate staffing is preferable to the risk and cost of poor quality of care.

Evidence-Based Nursing

There is a growing body of knowledge known as Evidence-Based Nursing (EBN) or Evidence-Based Practice (EBP), which defines and hastens the process of embedding the findings of nursing research into clinical practice. EBP advocates the integration of the conscientious use of *best evidence* in combination with a *clinician's expertise* as well as *patient preferences and values* to make decisions about the care provided to patients.

In the past, it has taken as long as 15-20 years for evidence from nursing research to translate into clinical practice, which means that the old practices continue at the risk of harm to patients even when better practices have been identified and accepted. For example, nurses continued to change intravenous dressings daily long after significant evidence indicated that this practice *increased* the rate of infection. To provide safer patient care, we need to shorten the gap between scientific evidence and clinical practice. EBP is an approach that helps us to do this.

"There's a way to do it better...find it." — *Thomas Alva Edison*

Performance Improvement and You

It is likely that *you* are involved in performance improvement initiatives as a leader. If not, get involved because you can make a difference for the patients, your colleagues and your organization. Find out what indicators are being monitored for your nursing unit and how often. Likewise, find out how the data is collected. Ask about the results, trends, and goals, and to what the results are compared. Are the results compared to any external benchmarks or best practices? What is being done to improve results? What is the trigger that signals the need to do a root cause analysis? What is a root cause analysis? Is investigation being conducted to find out how similar nursing units are getting better results for the same indicators? Are the excellent results from your nursing unit being communicated to the rest of the healthcare organization? How? Is someone writing an article for a nursing journal to communicate this good news and these excellent practices to the rest of the nursing world?

Safety through Communication

One final thought—as we have discussed, it is important that you communicate with the patient (and all stakeholders) in a clear manner. This is essential for patient safety. Is the patient too anxious to listen? Can the patient hear? Can the patient see? Can the patient read? Can the patient understand and comprehend? Are you taking the time to listen to the patient? Does the patient have a failing memory? What language does the patient use? Do you know how to get an interpreter if there is a language barrier?

Perhaps most important, how is information communicated to family members or caregivers who will provide care once the patient has left the hospital? Use words from the patient's vocabulary, not the medical vocabulary. Interpret what the doctor said if the patient does not understand the message. For example, "The doctor said my test was positive. Is that good or is that bad?" All of this is simple and basic. You, of course, know this "inside and out." It bears reflecting upon in the light of patient safety.

"The operation of a healthcare service depends upon a complex interaction between the patient, the environment in which care is provided and the people, equipment and facilities that deliver the care." — *Sir Liam Donaldson, British physician and author*

Conclusion

When we introduced the concept of being a great charge nurse in the beginning of this book, we did not explicitly define what that means. However, patient safety and error prevention is at the heart of being a great charge nurse. Health care is a complex environment with an ever-changing mix of variables that further complicate your ability to lead. That being said, each of us should remember daily to "first do not harm".

Personal Lessons

Reflections

- What processes on your unit lend themselves to errors?
- How many of these can be fixed with relative ease?
- Would those in positions of authority have any clue that these systems are broken and need fixing? If not, how could you communicate these safety issues?
- What is your role in patient safety and error prevention?
- How can organizations such as JCAHO or IHI help you in your job?
- Are you aware of EBP? Is this terminology used in your organization?

Things to Remember

- Patient safety is Job No.1 for you as charge nurse. It is *the* most important thing that nurses do.
- When systems and processes do not lend themselves to safe practice or have high potential for error, it is your responsibility to let someone know. Perhaps it is your supervisor or someone in the quality department.
- There are a number of resources at your fingertips. Utilize them and stay knowledgeable about current trends and issues.
- Be aware of clinical indicators that are being measured in your place of work. Check to see how your results compare to goals or benchmark performance.
- Are you aware of the impact to patient safety when technology changes are made in your place of work?

One day when you are in charge, Rhonda (an RN member of your team) approaches you and says, "I have called Dr. Lopez to tell him that Mrs. Jackson is having chest pains. He is rounding in the CCU right now and will be here in a few minutes." You note that the doctor arrives on your unit and goes promptly to the room of Mrs. Jackson. Dr. Lopez comes out of her room and states that he wants Mrs. Jackson transferred to CCU right away. You call CCU to arrange for a bed. You then inform Rhonda of the doctor's visit and his order to transfer Mrs. Jackson to CCU as soon as possible. You tell her that CCU is ready for the transfer and that she is responsible for giving report and transferring the patient, and for checking for other pending orders for Mrs. Jackson. Rhonda says, "OK."

Ten minutes go by and you are aware that Mrs. Jackson has not been transferred to CCU. You find Rhonda in another patient's room and she says she cannot do the transfer right away. You ask Shantel, who is sitting at the nurses station working on the computer, if she could transfer the patient. She tells you she is busy doing some charting. You see Anthony and Ellen standing in a corner talking. You ask if either of them could transfer Mrs. Jackson. They both say she is not their patient. You see two physicians at the desk who are asking to speak with you, but you decide you must leave your charge duties and transfer Mrs. Jackson yourself.

After you have completed the transfer you find Rhonda and tell her you have taken care of everything. Rhonda says, "I was going to do that in a minute. I didn't think it was that urgent." You say, "Oh, that's okay. I just wanted you to know that Mrs. Jackson is now in CCU."

You return to the desk to find that Shantel is still at the computer. Anthony and Ellen are still talking in the corner and there are several STAT orders that have not been taken care of. The unit secretary says that the doctors who had wanted to talk with you earlier wants you to call their offices right away to discuss why their orders never get followed correctly on this unit.

Review Questions:

- How does this story relate to patient safety?
- How did you miss out on providing good care in this situation? What could be done next time?
- What content from previous chapters comes to mind in this scenario?
- What expectations must be set for your team?
- How will you help your team understand the importance of the situation?
- What are five things you must do to improve communication on your unit?
- What are five ways to provide feedback to your team members with performance issues?
- What resources/tools may assist you in this situation?
- To whom do you report this kind of error? Dr. Lopez? Your supervisor? Risk management?

Resources & References

Terms & Acronyms

- **Benchmark**—A goal to be attained or a "stretch" goal. Benchmarks are used in quality improvement programs to encourage the improvement of care.
- **EBN/EBP**—Evidenced-Based Nursing or Evidenced-Based Practice is the conscientious, explicit and judicious use of current best evidence in making decisions about the care of patients.
- **National Patient Safety Goals**—These are specific clinical goals and objectives that are established and monitored by the Joint Commission on accreditation of Healthcare Organizations.
- **Root Cause Analysis**—A process used to find the underlying cause(s) of a problem or error.
- **Sentinel Event**—An unexpected occurrence involving death, serious physical or psychological injury, or the risk thereof. Serious injury specifically includes loss of limb or

function. Sentinel events signal the need for root cause analysis and correction.

Patient Safety in the News

Overworking Nurses has Adverse Effects on Patient Safety

July 9, 2004

A nationwide study co-authored by a Grand Valley State University nursing professor found that the long hours worked by hospital staff nurses may have adverse effects on patient safety.

Dr. Linda Scott, Grand Valley associate professor of nursing in the Kirkhof College of Nursing, said after studying the work habits of 393 hospital staff nurses, the research team found that nurses working more than 12.5 consecutive hours were three times more likely to make an error than nurses working shorter hours. Working overtime at the end of a shift also increased the risk of making an error.

The study, led by University of Pennsylvania nursing professor Dr. Ann Rogers will be published in the Journal of Health Affairs [July/August 2004]. The study was conducted by giving nurses logbooks to track hours worked, overtime, days off and sleep/wake patterns for 28 days. Participants were asked to describe errors or near errors that might have occurred during their work periods.

Participants reported 199 errors and 213 near errors during the data-gathering period. More than half the errors (58 %) involved medication administration; other errors included procedural errors (18 %), charting errors (12 %), and transcription errors (7 %).

Researchers found that most hospital nurses no longer work eight-hour day, evening or night shifts. Instead, they may be scheduled for 12-hour, 16-hour or even 20-hour shifts. Even when working extended shifts (over 12.5 hours), they were rarely able to leave the hospital at the end of their scheduled shift. All participants reported working overtime at least once during the data-gathering period

58

and one-third of the nurses reported working overtime every day they worked.

"Both the use of extended shifts (over 12 hours) and overtime documented in this study pose significant threats to patient safety," Rogers said. "In fact, the routine use of 12-hour shifts should be curtailed and overtime—especially overtime associated with 12-hour shifts—should be eliminated."

The study was funded with a grant from the Agency for Healthcare Research and Quality in Maryland. Scott and Rogers are conducting a correlating study to research the work hours of critical care nurses.

Scott and Rogers are expected to speak before their respective state legislatures on nurse fatigue and patient safety. Scott is also working with the Michigan Nurses Association on patient safety legislation.

"We need to educate nurses and hospitals about fatigue," she said. "It's a shared responsibility and both parties are accountable. This is a national problem and will likely have a national effect."

Reprinted with permission

Additional Resources

- Books
  - *Protect Yourself in the Hospital: Insider Tips for Avoiding Hospital Mistakes for Yourself or Someone You Love* by Thomas A. Sharon
  - *Evidence-Based Practice in Nursing & Healthcare: A Guide to Best Practice* by B. Melnyk and E. Fineout-Overholt (editors)
- Organizations
  - *National Patient Safety Foundation* (www.npsf.org)
  - *Joint Commission on Accreditation of Healthcare Organizations* (www.jcaho.org)

- US Department of Health and Human Services (www.hhs.gov)
  - Centers for Disease Control (www.cdc.gov)
  - Agency for Healthcare Research and Quality (www.ahrq.gov)
  - Centers for Medicare and Medicaid Services (www.cms.gov)
  - National Committee for Quality Assurance (www.ncqa.org)
  - World Health Organization (www.who.int/patientsafety)

- Journals
  - *Worldviews on Evidence-Based Nursing* (www.nursingsociety.org/publications)
  - *Evidence-Based Nursing* (ebn.bmj.com).

References

Aydin, C. E., Bolton, L. B., Donaldson, N., Brown, D. S., Buffum, M., Elashoff, J. D. & Sandhu, M. (2004). Creating and analyzing a statewide nursing quality measurement database. *Journal of Nursing Scholarship, 36*(4), 371-378.

IHI Launches National Campaign to Save 100,000 Lives in U.S. Hospitals (2005). *Psqh.com.* Retrieved December 14, 2013 from www.psqh.com/janfeb05/100k.html.

Institute of Medicine. (2000). *To err is human: Building a safer health system.* Washington, DC: National Academy Press.

The Leapfrog Group. Retrieved December 20, 2013 leapfroghospitalsurvey.org.

Joint Commission on Accreditation of Healthcare Organization's National Patient Safety Goals. *Jointcomission.org.* Retrieved December 10, 2013 from www.jointcommission.org/standards_information/npsgs.aspx.

Patient safety in the news: Overworking nurses has adverse effects on patient safety (2004). News-medical.net. Retrieved December 12, 2013 from www.news-medical.net/news/2004/07/09/3194.aspx.

Rosenstein, A. & O'Daniel, M. (2005). Disruptive behavior and clinical outcomes: Perceptions of physicians and nurses. *Nursing Management, 36*(1), 18-27.

Chapter Six
Patient Satisfaction & Service Recovery

"To provide appropriate service you have to know what your customer is feeling." — *Dan James, artist and author*

Until the early 1990s, not much thought was given to whether or not patients were satisfied. It was just assumed that they were doing okay, except for the occasional "complainer." I (Cathy) remember the first time I heard that the hospital where I worked would conduct standardized, periodic surveys of our patients to assess their level of satisfaction. I was the director of nursing, and was assigned lead responsibility for analyzing the results. I was not worried. I was confident the patients would give us great ratings. Alas, they did not! The scores were all over the place.

Health care was slower than other businesses—even other service industries—to study patient (customer) satisfaction. Looking back, it is hard to understand why, since now it is standard operating procedure to do these surveys and to act on the results. Perhaps it was related to the fact that physicians and nurses strongly objected to the notion of health care as a business and the identifying of patients as customers.

Several events, external to healthcare providers, took place in the last two decades of the 20th century that changed the way the healthcare industry behaved. The implementation of Diagnostic Related Groups (DRGs) had the potential to decrease hospital revenue. This risk caused healthcare organizations to look more carefully at their finances. DRGs caused hospitals to shorten lengths of stay. This action resulted in dissatisfaction for both patients and physicians. To maintain a healthy bottom line, healthcare organizations needed to increase the number of patients served per year to fill the beds that were opened up as lengths of stay decreased. However, it became apparent that the goal of efficiency had to be balanced with the goal of patient satisfaction.

During this same period of time, consumers became more educated and demanding, and the old patriarchal system in which patients went wherever their doctors directed began to break down. Patients began to make choices whenever it was within their power to do so. Likewise, physicians became less loyal to any one healthcare organization, taking their patients to the healthcare organizations where they thought their patients were most satisfied.

Additionally, mergers of healthcare systems began to occur which broke down the old system of independent community healthcare organizations. Healthcare systems negotiated with third party payers for preferred provider status. Third party payers began to request information about clinical outcomes *and* patient satisfaction in an attempt to swing business to the providers where people would not only receive the best clinical care but also be most satisfied.

Health care became more competitive and businesslike. Although painful, these changes have been positive in that they have caused the quality of care to improve. The changes have caused us to do what's right—not only to improve clinical care, but also to improve patient satisfaction. Today, patient satisfaction awareness is a part of our culture, and we are more interested in how we are perceived by patients. Needless to say leading your team to solid patient satisfaction scores will be an important part of your job.

"It is not the employer who pays the wages. Employers handle the money. It is the customer who pays the wages." — *Henry Ford, entrepreneur*

Lessons Learned

Due to increased focus on patient perceptions, the healthcare industry has studied and learned much about what satisfies (and dissatisfies) patients. Enough "big data" on this topic exists for the industry to draw some conclusions based on survey results, and to implement improvements. We have learned that meeting needs and exceeding patients' expectations is not easy. Satisfaction is more subjective than objective, and, therefore, better approaches are not so easy to design or implement.

To better understand the phenomenon of satisfaction, healthcare organizations and service industry experts study the customer satisfaction surveys of other types of businesses. However, the databases and resultant strategies on the topic of customer satisfaction from non-healthcare industries are somewhat dissimilar to those in health care. Think about it. No one chooses to be in a hospital or nursing home. The patients are virtual prisoners. We take their clothes, freedom of choice and dignity. They come to us not feeling well in the first place. Then, we poke and prod them, put them through unpleasant tests and procedures, and give them bad news ranging from tasteless diets to terminal diagnoses. Sometimes we speak an unfamiliar language and act hurried and uncaring. Patients and their significant others are anxious, frightened, angry and lonely. No wonder it is difficult to achieve high scores on patient satisfaction surveys.

Regardless of the challenges, we have learned that patient satisfaction is *not* a program. It is a change in philosophy. It is a change in the way we conduct ourselves each minute of the day. It works best when this change is systemic to the entire workplace. If we treat each other with dignity and respect, the entire culture becomes more caring and compassionate. Mutual respect is one of the most necessary ingredients in creating a healing environment— which, after all, is what nursing is all about.

We have also learned that in the minds of most patients, we are all responsible for each other's behaviors and actions. This means that patients really do not care *who* is to blame for what, they just know how they feel and they want problems fixed. If an inpatient has a bad time in the emergency department, the dissatisfaction experienced at the first point of contact can become a cloud of distrust and suspicion over the actions of all who care for the patient throughout their stay. If the discharge process does not go smoothly, this last moment of contact with the organization may cast a negative shadow over the memory of the entire experience. An environment in which patients are consistently satisfied requires leadership and proactive performance *all* the time. It requires that everyone be "tuned in" to the individual needs of others.

"Be everywhere, do everything, and never fail to astonish the customer." — *Motto of Macy's, department store*

Drivers of Patient Satisfaction

The accumulated data tells us that a few factors drive patient satisfaction. If these happen for the patients, they are more likely to feel satisfied with their stay. These factors are more qualitative than quantitative; more subjective than objective. They are common sense and yet in the busy, sometimes impersonal world of healthcare organizations, they do not consistently occur. The two professional groups that are drivers of satisfaction are physicians and nurses (especially nurses). This is not surprising since these are the two groups of professionals that patients associate with healthcare organizations. In the case of nurses, they are the group most frequently in contact with the patient. Many studiers of patient satisfaction cite *nurse communication* as the *factor with the greatest impact on patient satisfaction.*

Patients (and their families) want people to introduce themselves by name, explain why they are in the room and what they are about to do. They want *relationships* and *communication with nurses.* Also they want *information* and *education.* They want to know what is going on with their tests and what will happen next. They want to know which doctor is doing what. They want to feel like *partners* in their own care and plan of treatment. If they hear conflicting bits of information from different caregivers they want clarification. They want caregivers to have time for them and not appear to be rushed. Most of all, they want their nurses to be professional, warm, caring, and compassionate.

The Studer Group (www.studergroup.com) has done extensive work with healthcare organizations implementing methods to improve patient satisfaction. Studer has developed the acronym

AIDET that is helpful in remembering some basic satisfier behaviors:

- <u>A</u>cknowledge the patient and others in the room with a smile. Make eye contact and, if possible, sit down.
- <u>I</u>ntroduce yourself, your role/skill and experience.
- <u>D</u>uration—Go over length of time for tests, when to expect physician visits and other events.
- <u>E</u>xplanation—Describe step by step what will happen, answer questions, and explain how to reach a caregiver.
- <u>T</u>hank you—Is there anything else I can do for you?

"Perception is real even when it is not reality." — *Edward de Bono, leadership author*

Press Ganey (pressganey.com) is an independent organization that has surveyed millions of patients. Based upon the analysis of results, the group has summarized which factors are key in driving patient satisfaction.

Press Ganey Patients' Top Ten List

1. The staff responded to any inconvenience I had.
2. The hospital was cheerful.
3. The staff worked together to care for me.
4. The nurses responded to my concerns and complaints.
5. The staff was concerned about my comfort during tests and treatments.
6. The nurse kept me informed.
7. The staff addressed my emotional needs.
8. The staff included me in decisions.
9. The staff paid attention to my special or personal needs.
10. The staff tried to control my pain.

As you can see, many of these have a subjective quality to them. One reason patient satisfaction is often elusive is due to the fact that it is based more on perceptions and feelings than on facts.

Many hospitals use the Hospital Consumer Assessment of Healthcare Providers and Systems (HCAHP) Survey (www.hcahponline.org), also known as The Consumer Assessment of Healthcare Providers and Systems (CAHPS) Survey, to question patients about their healthcare experience. HCAHP provides a standardized survey instrument and data collection methodology for measuring patents' perspectives on hospital care. Since it is a standardized instrument that is used by many the results are comparable across hospitals. Results are publicly reported and available not only to third party payers, but also consumers of health care.

As a nurse leader you should learn as much as you can about the patient satisfaction process in your healthcare organization. What survey is used? What questions are asked? What are the trends in scores? What happens to subjective or unsolicited feedback such as written comments? What are the drivers that indicate repeat business or referred business for your healthcare organization? Are results available specifically for your department or unit? What initiatives have been implemented to improve scores—such as suggested scripts to help people say the right things at the right times? Can you join a committee or task force to help with these initiatives? Meet with the person in charge of patient satisfaction in your facility to learn the answer to these questions. They will appreciate your care and concern.

From a positive perspective, a complaint can be thought of as a gift. Patients see and experience the organization from a perspective that is fresh and different. When they verbalize complaints, patients are often providing valuable feedback. Addressing concerns allows patients to feel valued, respected and, therefore, better prepared to heal. Think of complaints as indicators for improvement. Thinking of them as irritants gets you nowhere.

"Customer complaints are the schoolbook from which we learn." — *Anonymous*

Sometimes the issue of improving patient satisfaction scores gets blown out of proportion. Administrators who do not take time to understand the complicated dynamics of patient care may focus only on the key drivers or the survey results. These individuals may think that, since the behaviors and actions of nurses are so important in determining patient satisfaction level, it must be nursing's fault when the scores are lower than desired. This can result in an undeserved heavy-handedness toward front-line caregivers. You may hear a rumor or a message like, "If satisfaction scores don't improve, something bad is going to happen. People will be disciplined and fired."

This, of course, creates a challenging environment. Nurses become afraid to do what is best for the patient because it may cause the patient to become dissatisfied. For example, a doctor orders a patient to get out of bed and sit in a chair for a couple of hours each shift. If the patient doesn't feel like getting out of bed and sitting up, the nurse may let the patient stay in bed out of fear of dissatisfying the patient. This is not good. If you see this happening, you need to talk about it in a staff meeting or with your supervisor. Get the issue out on the table. You can't let fear and rumors get in the way of your ultimate mission which is to providing good nursing care.

"Organizations have more to fear from lack of internal customer service than from any level of external customer service." — *Ron Tillotson, performance improvement author*

Contributing to Patient Dissatisfaction

Caregivers become so accustomed to their daily routine that they sometimes forget that it is all new and foreign to the patient, and that they need to take the time to explain everything—the environment, the daily schedule, who is doing what, and so forth. At times, nurses and other caregivers are so busy trying to be all things to all people that, to the patient, they don't appear to have the time to care or answer questions. It is a good habit to pause before you leave a patient's bedside, smile, take a breath and *sincerely* ask, "Is there anything else I can do for you? Do you have any questions? I have the time." The mere act of saying these words helps the patient relax and feel that you truly care.

Many people attend to the patient; many people go in and out of the room. And, although patients may think we are communicating with one another, often we are not. A patient may ask, "Who was that doctor who just came to see me? I have never met her before. And why was she here? She told me something about a test she was ordering. Can you explain that to me? She was in such a hurry I felt as though she didn't have time for my questions." You may not know the answer. To the patient this is a simple question; to you it is not. There is so much going on it is not possible for you to know everything. However, patients see you—especially in the role of charge nurse—as "all knowing." Saying "I don't know" is the wrong response; however, if those words are quickly followed with "but I will find out and get right back to you," you are on the road to meeting the patient's needs.

When other departments behave in a way that is dissatisfying to a patient (e.g., bringing the wrong lunch tray or delaying an X-ray) the patient's frustration is often vented on the nurse. If you respond by saying, "That's not nursing's fault; that is radiology's fault," this only causes the patient to become more frustrated. Skip over whose fault it is. Thank the patient for letting you know of the problem and then proceed to fix it. Later, explain to the patient what you have done about the complaint. It is *always* important to get back to a patient. It is satisfying to the patient if you bring closure to the communication loop.

Service Recovery: Addressing Patient Complaints

A small percentage of patients (and families) seem to be very rarely satisfied (maybe 5%). This is true inside and outside of healthcare organizations. Their cups are half empty. The best approach is for you and your team to develop a nursing plan of care that emphasizes a consistent approach.

On the flip side, there are a percentage of patients who are always sweet, pleasant, optimistic and forgiving. Only the worst of events

69

will cause them to be dissatisfied. They make up another five percent or so of the patient mix. It is the 90 percent in the middle who need that extra caring and communication to feel satisfied. It is this same 90 percent who give the most honest and helpful feedback in surveys.

The ideal approach to satisfying patients is to *do the job correctly the first time*. As legendary basketball coach John Wooden once said, "If you don't have the time to do it right the first time, when will you have the time to do it over?"

If patients feel satisfied and secure in the care they receive, they will likely be positive and accepting of every interaction. Unfortunately, this does not always happen. Consequently, nurses are placed in the position of s*ervice recovery* — trying to turn a negative or frustrating experience into a positive one. This takes more effort and consistency. The playing field is not level. The patient (and their families) may be anxious, watchful, fearful, doubtful, pessimistic and not as trusting as if all had gone well from the start.

As you know, as charge nurse, you will most likely get involved in service recovery. It may come to your attention that a patient or their significant others are upset. He or she has probably just said to the direct caregiver, "I want to speak to your supervisor." You are being given an opportunity to turn a difficult situation around. The good news is that if service recovery is successful, the result may produce a feeling of higher satisfaction in the patient than if the service failure had never occurred.

"Good judgment comes from experience. And where does experience come from? Experience comes from bad judgment."
— *Mark Twain, author*

Many nurses excel at service recovery. However, a small percentage of nurses may need coaching in this area. Brushing up on ways to turn service failure around will not only increase patient satisfaction but also increase nurse satisfaction. The feeling of *"what am I supposed to do now?"* will be replaced with *"I know what to do now."*

Until the steps of service recovery become second nature to you this is a perfect practice field for the "acting" we mentioned in Chapter One. It is important to know that there is usually only one chance to be "forgiven" for dissatisfying events. Therefore, it is helpful and important to be prepared with a formula to follow. The acronym **PLEASED** is one way to remember the steps of service recovery.

- **Promptly respond**. Act in a calm, courteous, professional manner. Address the patient as "Ms." or "Mr."
- **Listen actively, attentively and empathetically**. Clarify and ask questions. Repeat the story so that you and the patient agree as to the nature of the concern. Try to understand not only the facts, but also the patient's feelings. Make an empathetic statement such as, "I can see why you are frustrated." Be open and aware of your non-verbal communication, which can sometimes aggravate patients. Finally, do not be defensive and do not talk about who is at fault.
- **Express your apologies and own the responsibility for the service failure**. Say something like "I am sorry you are dissatisfied. I will correct that for you." This is a powerful statement. It acknowledges that the patient is not satisfied and that you will try to fix the problem. It does not mean you are guilty or at fault.
- **Agree to the next steps**. Explain to the patient what you are going to do and clarify expectations. If possible offer alternative approaches so that the patient regains control. For example, "I am going to call your physician right now with your questions. He usually responds within 30 minutes. If it is going to be longer than that I will tell you about how long it will be. Or I can give you his contact information and you can call him yourself. Which way is better for you?"
- **Seek resolution to the problem.** Act quickly. If you do not have time to investigate immediately and resolve the

issue, delegate it to someone who is reliable, accurate and quick. Keep the patient updated on your progress.

- **Explain the status or outcome to the patient as soon as there is resolution**. Go over step-by-step what you have done to fix the problem. If possible, explain that it is fixed in such a way that it will not happen to another patient and thank them for the feedback. This places the patient in the role of hero and erases any guilt he may feel for complaining. If there is no resolution when your shift is over, explain to the patient that you have to go home but that "Nurse Jane" is continuing to work toward resolution. If there is a barrier to fixing the issue, admit it. "I'm sorry, but radiology cannot do your test today because of several emergency patients. It will be done tomorrow. Are you OK with that?" Then ask, "Is there anything else that you need or that I can do for you."
- **Double check on the patient a little later and the next day to see how he or she is doing**. Convey your sincere apology again and communicate the message that you want the patient to have the best possible experience. Help the patient see you as an advocate. Thank the patient for bringing the situation to your attention.

The paradox of service recovery is that if it is done well it can result in a higher feeling of satisfaction than if the service failure had never occurred.

As charge nurse, your role in patient satisfaction may sometimes feel more demanding, complex and time consuming than the clinical aspects of the position. Think of it as an important part of your job. Develop the mindset that as charge nurse one of your roles is to foster and promote patient satisfaction.

As leader of the team you are seen as a role model. Be the compassionate caring nurse that you want others to be. Start first with seeing to the needs of team members. Are the needs of the caregivers being met? Do they have the resources and support required to feel safe and secure in doing their jobs? Are you thanking individuals for their good work? Be alert to disgruntled or low energy team members. Take a moment with these individuals to offer words of encouragement or to ask if they are OK. Let them know you are here for them. Often this is all it takes to get people back on the right track. If team members are happy it is likely that patients will feel more satisfied with their care.

In the course of your shift, take note of patients or significant others who indicate they have questions or concerns. Show interest in the person and the issues. Listen, repeat the concern for clarification, and act to fix the problem if you can. Try to understand what is behind the dissatisfaction. Is it really the stated facts or situation, or is there a deeper feeling like anxiety, loneliness or pain? Alert the nurse assigned to that patient. Come to an agreement on how to include measures in the plan of care that will better meet the communication or emotional needs of the patient.

Make it your daily goal to create an optimistic positive environment on your unit. If you achieve this objective, patients, caregivers, and all other stakeholders will feel more satisfied.

"Reality doesn't bite, rather our perception of reality bites."
— *Anthony D'Angelo, leadership author*

Personal Lessons

Reflections

- Has there been a time recently when you received poor customer service? Where were you? What problems did you experience?
- How did those serving you respond to your complaints or concerns? Was there a sincere apology or did it feel forced?
- Did you encounter systems problems (flawed processes) or personality problems?
- What are the most frequent complaints on your unit?
- Are the complaints due to personalities or broken systems?

- What service recovery training have individuals received on your unit?
- You should learn as much as you can about the patient satisfaction process used in your healthcare organization. What survey is used? What are the trends in scores? What happens to subjective or unsolicited feedback? Is this compiled and trended?

Things to Remember

- We have learned that patient satisfaction is *not* a program. It is a change in philosophy. It is a change in the way we conduct ourselves each minute of the day. It works best when this change is systemic. An environment in which patients are consistently satisfied requires everyone's commitment, *all the time.*
- Patients want people to introduce themselves by name, explain why they are in the room and what they are about to do. They want relationships and communication with nurses, information and education.
- As charge nurse, your role in patient satisfaction can be as demanding and complex as the clinical aspects of the position.
- Pay close attention to the perceptions of the patients with whom you are working. The more you can see things through their eyes, the more attentive you will be to their needs.
- Avoid fault-finding.
- A quick and effective service response can change a bad rating to a good one

The following **forbidden phrases** tend to inflame situations. What **acceptable phrase** could be used in its place?

Forbidden Phrase	**Correct Phrase**
"You'll have to…"	
"I'll have to…"	
"I don't know."	
"We can't do that."	
"You misunderstood me."	
"We are short staffed."	
"Hang on a second, I'll be back."	
"You should…"	
"That's not my fault."	
"I have no idea."	

Case Study—An Unforgettable Flight

Imagine you have never flown in an airplane, but tomorrow morning you will have to take your first flight with your five-year-old son across the country. You are nervous because you have never flown before. You are afraid of flying. You are nervous for your child's safety as well as your own. Images of that horrible story on the news race through your mind along with every movie that ever had a bad scene about airplanes. For some reason, that's all you can think about. Those with whom you have spoken brush off your fears and say, "It's safe. You'll be fine!"

Much to your dismay, the flight will take five hours, so you will have to wake up at least three hours before that (4 a.m.). The morning of the flight, there is a severe thunderstorm warning which does not help your mindset. Bravely, you make your way to the airport and prepare for your flight. After waiting 30 minutes in line, the first person you encounter is the baggage agent. She appears stressed out and is curt with you. She checks your bags and says, "Gate 17C, over there." Having never been in the airport, "over there" was not much help. Before you can ask a follow-up question, the man behind you is already checking in.

You wander around and find a sign for Terminal C. You move through security where they make you take off your shoes and pull you aside to search your carry-on luggage. They not only go through your things, but also frisk you and berate you for not taking off your belt. You ask why they are doing this and the agent responds, "It's the policy. They make us do this, ever since 9/11." Your child starts crying. Your anxiety level rises.

Finally, you arrive at your gate. Your flight is delayed. You wait in line for 15 minutes and ask the gate agent how long the delay will be. She looks at you and says, "It could be up to two hours. Can I do anything for you?" You respond, "No" and sit down. The gate area is packed with people. Children are crying and your son is becoming restless. The battery in the iPad is low and you cannot locate an outlet. Two hours turn into three. You look outside and notice that the storm has not subsided—in fact, the weather looks worse.

After one more hour, it is time to go. The agent mentions that some work needed to be done on the plane. Thoughts run through your head. What does this mean? Is this plane in need of repair? You want to call your husband but, by this time, you are being herded onto the plane. As you pass the cockpit, you see all kinds of buttons, lights and knobs. The pilots are working frantically and, as you are looking, the flight attendant interrupts and asks you to move along to your seat.

You stuff your carry-on into the overhead, sit down, and place all of your attention on taking care of your son. Because of this, you miss all the pre-flight instructions. A flight attendant comes by and snaps, "Ma'am put your tray table up and stow your purse. You are holding us up!" At this point, you want to cry. You look out the window at gray skies and rain. The engines begin. You hear strange noises. Finally, you are in the air. The majority of the flight is filled with turbulence. At one point, even the flight attendants have to sit down.

At long last, you land and as you are leaving the plane, the flight attendant says, "Hope you had a great flight! Come fly with us again!"

You can see where this quick story is going. The majority of patients you see every day are flying for the first time. For them, everything is stormy. They are worried about their children and family; they are worried about their safety. They do not understand the machines in the room. They do not understand clinical terminology (you might as well be speaking Latin) and they do not understand what is happening to their bodies. All they know is that they are on a flight they never wanted to take; however, they do know one thing—they know how they *feel*.

If they do not *feel* good, if things in the environment are aggravating them, if they do not understand, if they have had to wait a long time or if they perceive a negative attitude from an employee, you know the results. It is likely that as charge nurse, you will encounter people "on bad flights." Try to put yourself in their shoes, and try to view the situation from their point of view. They are scared. This will help you empathize and work through their issues. Often they just want to vent and know that you are there and you care. Finally, remember that family members are on the flight as well. They are also along for an unpleasant ride and, understandably, they are not at their best either.

Review questions:
- How do your organizational processes *contribute* to an individual's anxiety or apprehension?
- How do your co-workers *contribute* to an individual's anxiety or apprehension?
- Who in your organization best displays effective service recovery?
- What is your process for turning around a difficult situation with a patient?

Resources & References

Terms & Acronyms

- **DRGs**—Diagnosis Related Groups. A patient classification system that provides a way to describe types of patients. DRGs are the basis of the system used by Medicare to pay healthcare providers.
- **Service Recovery**—The redemptive actions that a provider takes in response to an actual or perceived service failure.
- **Third Party Payer**—Any payer for health care service other that the patient, for example, a health insurance company or Medicare.

Additional Resources

- *Knock Your Socks Off Service Recovery* by Ron Zemke & Chip R. Bell
- *Resolving Patient Complaints*: *A Step-By-Step Guide to Effective Service Recovery* by Liz A. Osborne
- *If Disney Ran Your Hospital, 9 1/2 Things You Would Do Differently* by Fred Lee
- *Resolving Complaints for Professionals in Health Care* by Wendy Leebov
- *Resolving Patient Complaints: A Step-By-Step Guide* by Liz Osborne

Chapter Seven
Mentoring Your Staff

"Treat people as if they were what they ought to be and you help them become what they are capable of being." — *Eudora Welty, author and photographer*

Just as you have mentors, you can mentor others. In fact, great leaders are known for developing other great leaders. Nurses have often been accused of "eating their young." This is a phrase we could do without. We need to do a better job of coaching and mentoring each other. We all know that it is difficult to "hang in there" as a nurse. It is even harder for a new nurse or a nurse new to an environment.

Many institutions have formal mentoring programs and some do not. Regardless, in the role of charge nurse, there is plenty of opportunity to coach and mentor. Be a hero. When you are in charge, take time to consider the people who are in need of mentoring. Try to remember what it has been like for you and put yourself in the new team member's shoes. Do for them what was done for you (or what you wish had been done for you).

Painful experiences that occur during orientation remain memories for a long time. The first time I (Cathy) passed medications on my first job is one such memory for me. I was partnered with an experienced nurse who was focused on my progress. This part of the memory is good. I felt that my performance was a priority for her and that she was taking seriously the responsibility of teaching me on the job. On the 8 a.m. medication rounds, I had a "near miss." A patient was scheduled for surgery and I failed to note this in her orders. I almost medicated her, but caught the error in time. At the end of the day, the nurse assigned to orient me told me that she thought I had made a mistake in choosing the profession of nursing. She berated me for my inattention to detail and accused me of having an uncaring attitude toward patients. This was devastating and I will never forget her words. Her coercive approach worked in that I was determined to do a better job; however, it also left me with a sour taste and I was determined to be an encouraging and positive mentor to others. Learning through fear and intimidation is ineffective. A good mentor inspires trust and confidence.

Almost every day that you are in charge you will be given the opportunity to coach and mentor: brand new nurses, experienced new hires, floats, per diem nurses, new charge nurses, new managers, new people in other departments, residents, fellows and new physicians. First you need to get out of the mindset that mentoring takes hours and hours of time. In reality, it may be a five second interaction or three minute tutorial. Healthcare organizations hire many people and every month there is a new batch of protégés. Wouldn't it be great if they stayed with the organization for a long time? It would decrease the shortage of workers and eliminate the feeling that "everyone around here is so new they don't quite know what they are doing."

"I know of no more encouraging fact than the unquestionable ability of man to elevate his life by conscious endeavor."
— *Henry David Thoreau, author, poet and philosopher*

The Cost of Poor Mentoring

Organizations spend thousands of dollars to hire each nurse. It is expensive to recruit registered nurses because they are highly skilled professionals and they are scarce. It is also estimated that as many as 50 percent of new hires leave within the first six months *if they do not receive a solid orientation*. It is only at the end of six months that employees can begin to be as productive as an experienced worker. It takes even longer than six months for nurses, particularly specialty nurses, to be self-sufficient. So, you can see that millions of dollars would be saved if we retained nurses.

However, that is not the most important reason to coach, mentor and retain nurses. The *standard of care* in any healthcare organization is directly related to the expertise and tenure of its nurses. Excellent nurses who have worked together over time deliver world-class care. If excellent nurses are retained, patient care is exceptional.

It seems so easy to understand. It is so logical. And yet, it is difficult to find a healthcare organization where nurse orientation and mentoring is given the high priority it deserves. Each of us must be the best mentor we can be to help each nurse reach his or her potential as a clinician and as a team member.

"Two hallmarks that distinguish the good mentor from the mediocre teacher are recognition that passion is central to learning and the capacity to provide emotional support when it is needed." — *Stephen Brookfield, educator*

Mentoring Takes Time (But Not As Much As You Think)

Wherever you work, it is likely that there is an orientation program with a plan and a process that is tailored to every protégé. The barrier to carrying out these plans is usually finding the time. The key component to effective coaching and mentoring is *quality* time. However, setting aside time for the required communication and attention is given low priority in the crunch to get everything done. It is even sometimes difficult to consistently pair a new nurse with the same person day after day. Schedules and other responsibilities cause the orientation plan to get lost in the shuffle, which may cause the new nurse to feel personally lost, alone and dissatisfied.

There is no easy fix for the dilemma of the time crunch that is felt by all health care providers in healthcare organizations. Regardless, mentoring *must* be a priority and can be accomplished in small, bite-sized chunks. Guiding the professional development of a new nurse is definitely a wonderful way to spend your time. It is the opportunity to pass along the wisdom, caring and confidence you have earned. The most magical gift you can give is to nurture a supportive and encouraging relationship with the person you are mentoring.

81

There is a phenomenon known as the *Pygmalion Effect*. You are probably familiar with it. It is a performance-stimulating effect. People who are led to expect that they will do well, will do better than those who expect to do poorly, or do not have any expectations about how well or how poorly they will do (Bass, 1985). Mentors who arouse in protégés confidence in their abilities will increase the likelihood of their success. When a mentor devotes time to the experience and expresses satisfaction, praise and encouragement, the protégé is more likely to do well. A positive, accepting and supportive relationship with a protégé is likely to result in developing a positive, confident and caring nurse.

"My chief want in life is someone who shall make me do what I can." — *Ralph Waldo Emerson, author, poet and philosopher*

Characteristics of a Good Mentor

Experience has shown that effective nurse mentors have a positive attitude and are good at building caring relationships. They tend to be good listeners and are comfortable giving honest and constructive feedback. Good mentors are role models and are generous in providing moral support, guidance and encouragement. They enjoy the process of developing the skills and confidence of others. They are knowledgeable in the process of adult learning and provide appropriate levels of challenge *and* support.

Benefits for the Mentor

Experience has also shown that a positive mentoring relationship has many benefits for mentors. Mentors develop meaningful personal relationships and find new professional colleagues. The personal and professional growth and self-awareness received by protégés are mirrored in mentors. They gain satisfaction and learning intrinsic to the teacher-student relationship. Mentors are stimulated to question and improve their own nursing practice.

Not everyone likes to orient or train new people. It may not be enjoyable if you are untrained in mentoring techniques or do not have a genuine passion for mentoring. People who volunteer to be mentors do the best job at mentoring because of this passion and personal interest.

"If learning is about growth, and growth requires both trust and agency, then teaching is about recognizing and nourishing the conditions in which trust and agency can flourish. Teaching is thus preeminently an act of care." — *Larry Daloz, author on teaching and mentoring*

Improving Your Unit's Formal Mentoring Program

Russell and Adams (1997) define mentoring as an "interpersonal exchange between a senior experienced colleague (mentor) and a less experienced, junior colleague (protégé) in which the mentor provides support, direction and feedback regarding career plans and personal development" (p. 2). In addition, "mentors are frequently characterized as individuals who are committed to providing support to junior members in an effort to remove organizational barriers and to increase the upward mobility of their protégés" (p. 2).

According to Scandura, *et al.* (1996), research has shown that protégé promotions and compensation appear to be influenced by a mentor. Moreover, Forret *et al.* (1996) note that mentors provide protégés with career functions such as how to maneuver organizational politics. They also provide protégés with psychosocial functions, which increase their competence, effectiveness and work-role identity.

In their article *Making Mentoring Work*, Tabborn, Macaulay, & Cook (1997) discuss four key factors that make mentoring work: 1) a clear, agreed upon set of objectives; 2) communication and training; 3) matching of mentors and protégés; and 4) evaluation and review of the program. First, the unit needs to have a clear picture of how and why the mentoring program will be utilized. How will the mentoring program assist the unit in meeting its objectives? A clear definition, along with the support of unit mentors, will form a solid foundation for the program. Second, unit leaders will need education on the process of mentoring and they will need a clear understanding of their role in the process. What are their objectives and expectations? What is their time commitment? All of these questions need to be answered. Further, mentors should be briefed (at least) in techniques of active listening, facilitation and base-line skill building. Third, the process for matching mentors with protégés should be thought through in a careful manner. There are a number of methods, and no one process has an overarching stamp of approval. Regardless of the process, the unit should be aware of how the method will affect mentors as well as protégés. Finally, units must evaluate and review their progress. Not only will this process assist the unit in determining success of the program, it will also assist unit leaders in evaluating the effect on the protégé.

Personal Lessons

Reflections

- Who are *your* mentors? If the process does not exist formally within your healthcare organization, seek individuals you respect and ask them if they would like to have lunch once a month. In addition, remember that you may have a *network* of people you turn to for various needs. For instance, there may be someone you respect for his ability to lead change while another person may be a great at building teams.

Things to Remember

- Mentoring is one of the most important roles an individual can play within a unit. Helping someone acclimate to co-workers and equipment is an important role because it defines and shapes a new team member's initial impressions of the unit and of the organization.
- Structure your mentoring program in a way that everything is spelled out. What are the expectations of the mentor? How about the protégé? How long will the relationship last?

- Good mentoring relationships are built on trust, allowing protégés the opportunity to build confidence in the process. Choose mentors who will take this commitment seriously.

Case Study—Your Organization's Culture

It is not unusual to feel that the mentoring or orientation program on your unit has always been a little weak. Maybe it's because mentoring is regarded as a mandate from the staff development department. Maybe it's because everyone is so busy that it is "just one more thing." Maybe it is because no one sees value in the activity. There are likely multiple reasons.

If you see the importance of a strong mentoring program you may have done a little extra reading or taken a continuing education class on the topic. You may be excited about what you have learned and wonder if the mentoring program on your unit could be improved. You may have done some research online and read articles about successful mentoring programs in health care. The ideas look *really* good and you see how your unit could benefit from them.

You are pretty sure that some of your friends at work would be interested in reading the articles and talking about them. You have a good rapport with your supervisor and you think he or she might be interested, too. You are not sure how to proceed. You begin to think about the current mentoring program.

Review Questions:

- What is successful about the mentoring program on your unit?
- What aspects are not successful?
- What barriers are getting in the way of a successful program?
- How do nurses become mentors? Do they volunteer or are they assigned to the role?
- Who are the best mentors on your unit? Why?
- Do they receive education on how to be mentors?

- Are they recognized for their efforts?
- Are clear expectations written for mentors and protégés?
- Based on what you have learned in this chapter what would you change or keep about your mentoring program?
- Who needs to be involved in revamping a mentoring program? What resources are available to assist you?

Resources & References

Terms & Acronyms

- **Mentor**—An individual or network of individuals who can help a Protégé learn about self, department or organization.
- **Mentoring Program**—A formal set of policies and procedures that guide a mentor/protégé relationship.
- **Mentoring Agreement**—An outline of objectives and guiding principles for the mentor/protégé relationship.
- **Protégé**—Usually a "junior" individual interested in learning from "senior/experienced" mentor.

Additional Resources

- *Mentoring Leaders: Wisdom for Developing Character, Calling, and Competency* by Carson Pue
- *The Handbook of Mentoring at Work: Theory, Research, and Practice* by Belle Rose Ragins
- *Coaching and Mentoring: How to Develop Top Talent and Achieve Stronger Performance* (Harvard Business Essentials) by Harvard Business School Press)
- *A Game Plan for Life: The Power of Mentoring* by Don Yaeger

References

Bass, B. (1985). *Leadership and performance beyond expectations*. New York: Free Press.

Forret, M. F., Turban, D. B., & Dougherty, T. W. (1996). Issues facing organizations when implementing formal mentoring programs. *Leadership & Organization Development Journal, 17*(3), 28-31.

Kohn, L., Carrigan, J. M., & Donaldson, M. S. (1999). *To err is human: Building a safer health system.* Institute of Medicine. Washington, D.C.: National Academy Press.

Mullich, M. (2004). They're hired: Now the real recruiting begins.*workforce.com.* Retrieved December 24, 2013 from www.workforce.com/articles/theyre-hired-now-the-real-recruiting-begins.

Reeves, K.A. (2004). Nurses nurturing nurses: A mentoring program. *Nurse Leader, 2*(6), 47-49.

Russell, J. & Adams, D. (1997). The changing nature of mentoring in organizations: An introduction to the special issue on mentoring in organizations. *Journal of Vocational Behaviors, 51*, 1-14.

Scandura, et al. (1996). Perspectives on mentoring. *Leadership and Organization Development Journal, 17*(3), 50-56.

Squires, A. (2004). A dimensional analysis of role enactment of acute care nurses. *Journal of Nursing Scholarship, 36*(3), 272-278.

Tabborn, A., Macaulay, S., & Cook, S. (1997). Making mentoring work. *Training for Quality, 5*(1), 6-9.

Chapter Eight
Delegation

Delegation is an essential skill for a charge nurse. At times, you must hand off the work to team members to simply get everything done. Delegation comes easily to some nurses but not to others. As young leaders develop and gain experience, they better understand their responsibility to delegate. Likewise, they begin to understand the nuances of being *members* of the team and *leaders* of the team. They understand that everyone is busy and that adding more work to a person's load is not to be done without thought and good reason. The first response of new leaders may be to try to do most of the work themselves. This is true for several reasons. First, they are trying to spare their colleagues additional work. Another reason is that, because they are truly excellent at what they do, they struggle because they may feel they are more effective and efficient than other members of the team.

"The surest way for an executive to kill himself is to refuse to learn how, and when, and to whom to delegate work." — *J.C. Penney, entrepreneur*

The breakthrough happens when it becomes obvious that it is not a reasonable plan to do all the work oneself. This realization comes quickly for charge nurses—within the first few hours of assuming the role! In the end, it is a leader's responsibility not only to delegate to get the work done efficiently, but also to create a team, engender trust, and *develop* the knowledge skills and abilities of the team. The effective leader learns how fairly distribute additional work assignments. She also learns how to help team members assimilate into their work plan additional tasks. This is part of developing individual team members.

Learning how to effectively delegate may take practice and experience, but your efforts will pay off for the team and the patients in the long run. You know you have arrived when you can go away for two weeks and, even in your absence, the floor clips along because you have helped build a cohesive and high functioning team.

As with most things, there is an art and a science to delegation. The *art* has to do with interpersonal communication and team-building skills. The *science* has to do with legal and licensure issues for registered nurses.

"Surround yourself with the best people you can find, delegate authority, and don't interfere."—*Ronald Reagan, 40th President of the United States*

The Art of Delegation

The art of delegation requires that you make the request tactfully, and that you remember to say "please" and "thank you" when you ask someone to take on extra tasks. Successful delegation will result in the team feeling strong and capable while unsuccessful delegation causes the team to feel overworked and victimized. Here are a few suggestions:

- *Delegate to the right person.* Be fair and don't always delegate to the same person. Keep track of how much everyone is already doing and try not to overload any one individual. Spread the tasks around.
- *Delegate the objective, not the procedure.* Outline the desired results, not the steps in the process (unless someone wants this). Team members may feel micromanaged if you tell them not only what to do, but also how to do it.
- *Clarify expectations.* Make sure the person to whom you delegate understands the ultimate objective and has a clear timeline for completion.
- *Check-in.* While in process, ask if the person needs additional resources to complete the task. Check to see how s/he is doing. This gives you assurance that the task is being completed. If done tactfully it communicates respect and back up to the person performing the task. If done poorly it may communicate lack of trust.

- *Express gratitude.* Say "thank you" at the time you delegate the task and again upon completion.

"You can delegate authority, but not responsibility."
— *Stephen W. Comiskey, leadership author*

The Science of Delegation

Delegation is addressed in the *American Nurses Association Code of Ethics for Nurses* (www.nursingworld.org/codeofethics). Once you are licensed as a registered nurse you are accountable for knowing and living by this code. The American Nurses Association (ANA) defines delegation as: "the transfer of responsibility for the performance of an activity from one person to another while retaining accountability for the outcome" (Principles for Delegation, 2005, p. 4).

The act of delegation is clarified in the Nurse Practice Act of the state in which you are licensed (www.ncsbn.org/4319.htm). You need to be familiar with these rules and regulations. Your daily actions must be consistent with the *Scope of Practice* as defined in the *Nurse Practice Act* that governs your professional practice and your work setting. Usually these concepts are incorporated into the job descriptions and policies and procedures of your organization.

You must take the time to acquaint yourself with the way delegation is expressed in your state's *Nurse Practice Act*. Take a continuing education course on delegation and ask your supervisor about it. Once you are familiar with the expectations and requirements, you will feel much more comfortable with the legal aspects of delegation.

"Words have the power to destroy or heal. When words are both true and kind, they can change the world." — *Buddha, spiritual leader, 560-480 BC*

Be sure to clarify the specific process of delegation within your facility, but some general thoughts are warranted.

Prior to delegation, the charge nurse must be knowledgeable of several aspects of care. With experience, this process becomes automatic or second nature, but it is good to be aware that this is what you are assessing before delegating.

1. Clinical assessment of the patient who needs nursing care.
2. Review of the assessments performed by other healthcare professionals.
3. Complexity and frequency of the nursing care needed.
4. Training, ability and skill required of the person to whom you will delegate.
5. Availability and accessibility of resources.

Delegation can also be seen as *Five Rights*.

1. *Right task*—The task is delegable and is for a specific patient.
2. *Right circumstance*—There is an appropriate patient setting, available resources, and consideration of other relevant factors.
3. *Right person*—The right person is delegating the right task to the right person to be performed on the right patient.
4. *Right direction/communication*—Delegation includes a clear, concise description of the task including objectives, limits and expectations.
5. *Right supervision*—Appropriate monitoring, evaluation, intervention and feedback are provided.

Finally, the ANA (http://www.nursingworld.org) states that there are three tasks that can only be done by or delegated to an RN.

1. The initial nursing assessment and any subsequent assessments or nursing interventions that require specialized nursing knowledge, judgment and skill.

2. The determination and formulation of the nursing diagnoses.
3. The identification of nursing care goals, development of the nursing plan of care in conjunction with the patient and/or family and evaluation of the patient's progress, in relation to the plan of care.

A Personal Story

Something happened to me (Cathy) early in my role as charge nurse that illustrates the need to be clear about what can be delegated to whom. A nursing assistant approached me and volunteered to start intravenous lines. She explained that she had been a phlebotomist before becoming a nursing assistant and that she was good at "difficult" starts. She further stated that she knew that hospital policy prevented her from performing IV starts, but she was willing to overlook that policy if I was. This was a tempting offer since it is not easy to find someone to start IV lines when the start is tricky and the line is needed right away. From a practical point of view, it probably would have been safe and relatively painless for the patient given the nursing assistant's previous experience. However, from a professional standpoint, the offer had to be declined given the hospital policy and the state board of nursing's position statement on intravenous lines.

In Closing

Delegation is a core function of effective leadership. Delegation must be based upon professional nursing judgment, state law and organizational policies. The guiding principles to consider when you delegate are as follows:

- *Legality*—the delegated task is within the scope of practice and not prohibited by law.
- *Competency*—the delegated task maintains standards of safe practice and the person to whom the delegation is made can demonstrate and document knowledge, skills and ability.

- *Safety*—the delegated task is safe and appropriate for the patient at this time.
- *Accountability*—the person to whom the delegation is made can perform according to standards of safe care and can accept accountability for nursing actions.
- *Respectfulness* - the person to whom the delegation is made should be addressed and acknowledged in a tactful and respectful manner.

Personal Lessons

Reflections

- When someone delegates a task to you, how do you like to be approached?
- When you have completed a task, how do you like to be recognized?
- What are some creative ways to follow up with people to be sure a task has been completed?
- How do you feel about delegation? Do you feel comfortable delegating tasks to others? Why or why not based on what we have discussed?
- What do you say or do when you delegate a task to someone and the response is "I am already swamped."

Things to Remember

- Delegation is an essential skill for charge nurses. Trying to do it all on your own simply will not work.
- Great leaders see themselves as *members* of the team. At times, they may need to assume control, but more often than not, they are simply the coordinator, making sure that everything functions well.
- There is an *art* and a *science* of delegation. The *art* has to do with interpersonal communication and team-building skills. The *science* has to do with legal and licensure issues for registered nurses. Observe how others around you practice the art and the science. Imitate those who do well

and avoid the approaches of those who are ineffective. Eventually, your own style will emerge.

Case Study—Vanetta

Vanetta Jackson, RN, is the charge nurse. It is a crazy day. The lab reports are late. The physicians are all arriving on the unit for rounds at the same time—right after their 7:00 a.m. staff meeting. There are several new physician orders that need to be initiated. Six discharge orders are among them. Admitting has called with five new admissions. ICU has called with a transfer. A physician is requesting assistance with the patient in room 536. There are 30 beds on the unit and all of them are occupied. It is 8:30 a.m. and time to send half of the staff on their morning breaks. On duty are:

- Lucy Silver, RN—an orienteer who is new to this unit, but a seasoned nurse
- Ann Davids, RN—six years' experience on this unit
- Will Allen, RN—agency nurse with seven years' experience
- Faith Plusek, LPN—20 years' experience on this unit
- George Leeming, NA—four years' experience on this unit
- Beatrice Talison, NA—25 years' experience on this unit

Lucy is not returning to the unit after break because she has to go to a class for orientation. The unit secretary called in sick and the staffing office cannot send anyone to cover. The ICU patient has to be transferred to the unit ASAP because the OR has a fresh post-op ready to go to ICU and there are no open critical care beds. In addition, one patient needs to be given intravenous antibiotics. The IV line has to be started and someone has to go to the pharmacy to get the antibiotic because the delivery system is not working. A family member is standing at the desk and wants someone to call her mother's physician. Vanetta has just been reminded that it is time to go to discharge planning rounds.

Review Questions:

- What would you do if you were Vanetta?
- Which tasks can she delegate and to whom?
- Which of these tasks should she do herself?
- How should she prioritize what needs to be done?
- Is there any way she can get more help?

Resources & References

Terms & Acronyms

- **Accountability**—To be accountable is to accept responsibility, liability and answerability for ones actions.
- **Code of Conduct**—A formal statement of the values and business practices of an organization, an entity or a professional group.
- **Delegation**—Delegation occurs when a leader or manager employs the assistance of others in completing common tasks that will benefit the patient or the unit.
- **Nursing Judgment**—Nursing judgment is the intellectual process that an RN exercises in forming an opinion and reaching a conclusion by analyzing the data.

Additional Resources

- *Making Delegation Happen: A Simple and Effective Guide to Implementing Successful Delegation* by Robert Burns
- *The Busy Manager's Guide to Delegation (Worksmart Series)* by Richard Luecke
- *Nursing Delegation and Management of Patient Care* by Kathleen Motacki
- *Delegation of Nursing Care* by Patricia Kelly-Heidenthal and Maureen Marthaler
- *Delegating Work (Pocket Mentor)* compiled by Harvard Business School Press

References

American Nurse's Association Code of Ethics for Nurses. Retrieved from http://www.nursingworld.org/codeofethics on December 1, 2013.

American Nurses Association (2005). Principles for Delegation. Washington, DC: American Nurses Publishing.

How to Delegate. Retrieved from http://getmoredone.com/2010/08/how-to-delegate/ on December 23, 2013.

Nursing Standards & Delegation: A Guide to Ohio Board of Nursing Rules. Ohio Board of Nursing – Laws and Rules. Retrieved from www.nursing.ohio.gov/Law_and_Rule.htm on December 14, 2013.

Chapter Nine
Leading through Conflict

Taking charge of a patient care unit in a healthcare organization provides all the ingredients for conflict. As the leader, you have the opportunity to prevent and manage conflict. This is an exciting and challenging part of your role. Here's where you demonstrate your best interpersonal skills, your powers of negotiation, your ability to influence and your intense focus on the patients.

There are different types of conflicts. The ability to recognize two types of conflict is helpful in finding resolution. Is the conflict *internal* or *external*?

"A real leader faces the music even when he doesn't like the tune." — *Anonymous*

Internal Conflict

An *internal* conflict exists within *you* and is usually the easiest type to resolve. For example, you may feel the urge to lash out but, instead, you must smile and be polite. Getting beyond internal conflict requires emotional intelligence, self-awareness, and maturity. It challenges you to choose your battles. Sometimes you have to learn the hard way. Here's an example. I (Cathy) used to work with a physician who was very dramatic and verbal when it came to expressing her frustration. In my first few encounters with her, I kept trying to move the conversation beyond the phase of venting to the stage of communicating information, explanations and problem-solving. This, I learned, only prolonged the volume and length of the venting phase. I learned that I needed to listen attentively and wait patiently until the doctor had calmed down enough to converse. The conflict was really within me—it was *internal*. I had to learn how to prevent escalation of the situation by controlling my reaction.

Internal conflicts usually involve strong feelings within you and require you to control not only verbal, but also non-verbal behavior. Sighing, rolling your eyes or folding your arms defiantly across your chest will only prolong and exacerbate the conflict.

"Whenever you're in conflict with someone, there is one factor that can make the difference between damaging your relationship and deepening it. That factor is attitude."
— *Timothy Bentley, leadership author and coach*

External Conflict

External conflict is either *situational* or *interpersonal*.

Situational conflicts are often temporary and exist in the moment. They often have to do with limited resources or incompatible priorities. For example, there is a last minute request for one of the nurses on your team to accompany her assigned patient to radiology. This request coincides with her assigned lunch break. At the same time, a new admission (which has been pre-assigned to her) arrives on the unit. The external conflict is that the nurse needs to be in three places at once. She may figure this out in collaboration with her teammates; however, it is possible that she will come to you for help in reallocating the workload. At the very least, she needs your approval to shift the work. Checking in with you (the charge nurse) is important so that you always know who is taking care of whom, who is off the unit, and so forth. If *situational* conflicts are resolved quickly and objectively, they usually do not escalate. One way of handling this type of situation is to make a decision in collaboration with team members which is based on data, to announce the decision and explain your reasons and then to move forward. You often do not have time for negotiation or a more democratic process.

"Whoever has the mind to fight has broken his connection with the universe. If you try to dominate people you are already defeated. We study how to resolve conflict, not how to start it."
— *Daniel Goleman, author*

The most difficult type of conflict to resolve is *interpersonal*. *Interpersonal* conflicts often occur in the work place and are an inevitable byproduct of human interaction, especially in the highly complex environment of health care. When an interpersonal conflict escalates, it is disruptive and distractive to patient care.

Conflict may result when there are differing goals, opinions or interpretations of roles and priorities. There may be an ongoing struggle for power or control that exists between two people or even factions. What turns these conflicts into unacceptable organizational upheaval are the strong emotions and inappropriate behavior that may accompany them.

As charge nurse you may witness a struggle between interdependent caregivers who perceive incompatible goals, scarce resources, and interference in achieving their goals. An effective leader recognizes an interpersonal conflict that is beginning to get out of control and acts quickly to redirect attention back to the work at hand. At best, this is an opportunity for personal and organization growth.

"In one's family, respect and listening are the source of harmony." — *Buddha, spiritual leader, 560-480 BC*

Be Alert to Potential Conflict

You get to know the people you work with and their personality traits, strengths and areas of growth. After a while, you can predict who will become involved in conflict and who will not. When you come on duty and are preparing for a shift, you learn to assess who is working with you and how they are feeling. Gauging the atmosphere and knowing the personalities helps you to be prepared.

Key observations may include: What are the group dynamics? Is there light-heartedness and are people quietly and cooperatively going about their work? Or, is there a feeling of sarcasm, anger, hostility and burnout? Even worse, is there complete silence? Can you "cut the air with a knife?" Calling this to people's attention at shift report may help. "What's going on? Everyone seems distracted." Get it out and talk about it. Remind everyone to focus on the patients and encourage everyone to work as a team. If it is necessary, pull people aside and discuss the situation. Ask for the team's cooperation in setting a positive tone. Help everyone to realize the need to get beyond whatever is causing the problem. Set a positive tone and move forward.

"In dwelling, live close to the ground. In thinking, keep to the simple. In governing, don't try to control. In work, do what you enjoy. In family life, be completely present." — *Lao-Tzu, Chinese philosopher, 604 BC*

Coping Skills

Leaders who excel at conflict prevention and management see conflict as an opportunity for growth. They read situations quickly and take responsibility for intervening. They are skilled at active listening, negotiating agreements and settling disputes equitably. They are good at quickly identifying common ground. They work toward gaining cooperation and trust from the parties involved in the conflict. They seek options and alternative strategies. These leaders focus on mutual respect, professionalism and finding the best solution for all involved. They encourage cooperation and help everyone to move on.

"Difficulties are meant to rouse, not discourage. The human spirit is to grow strong by conflict." — *William Ellery Channing, founder of Unitarianism*

If you find yourself faced with a conflict between two or more of your team members, you must act. Time spent involved in conflict is time spent away from patient care. You do not have a lot of time to waste and time will be wasted if you do not act. Resolving conflict takes courage, especially the first few times you do so. However, you gain confidence, skill and respect each time you act in the role of a fair mediator. *Once people realize you will address conflict, they will be less likely to engage in it.*

There are a few basics to remember when you are in the position of having to calm the emotions caused by interpersonal conflicts. You may not resolve the issues between entrenched enemies or dedicated troublemakers, but it is your job to get the team back on track. Most workplace conflict is not caused by perennial "bad actors" but is caused by well-meaning, focused people whose emotions and tempers flare up when they find themselves under stress and immersed in the two types of conflict previously discussed.

The first task is to determine if it is best to sit back and let people work it out for themselves or whether it is time for you to act. The scale of the disruption and the intensity of emotion will help you make this decision. With time and experience this will become easier.

Once you have chosen to intervene, it is important to approach the scene and then calmly and professionally assume the role of negotiator or intermediary. Ask the parties to calm down and lower their voices. Move parties to a private area if possible. Remember that everyone is watching and listening. Getting out of the spotlight really helps combatants remember where they are.

First, talk about the importance of getting back to work. State that you are there to help the parties arrive at some mutually acceptable compromise or resolution.

Next, ask what is going on. Ask for facts. Discourage accusations and emotional outbursts. Listen attentively and respectfully. Identify the common ground (e.g., efficient and effective patient care). Ask each party to allow the other to state their side of the argument without interruption. Summarize the conflict, as you understand it. Acknowledge the value of each point of view. Help everyone to maintain dignity.

Finally, ask each participant to suggest a resolution. Consider compromises. If participants cannot agree then it is your responsibility to decide on a plan. Request the participants to accept the plan. Thank them for participating in the conversation.

Then remind them that it is time to move on and focus on patient care.

The step-by-step approach described above is an extreme move. You rarely need to go through all of these steps—people just don't have time for it. They often come to their senses and realize they have to get beyond the conflict. Chances are you will reach a resolution much faster and with much greater ease than the above scenario suggests.

"The gem cannot be polished without friction, nor man perfected without trials." — *Confucius, Chinese philosopher, 551-479 BC*

A compounding factor is that one of the participants in a conflict may be a physician. All of the above suggestions still hold. There may be a perceived imbalance of power and inappropriate comments may occur in the heat of the conflict. Take charge. The patient's well-being is at risk. It has been my experience (Cathy) that if you act quickly, fairly and professionally, the doctor will be appreciative of your intervention. Just as you know which physicians are most likely to become embroiled in non-productive spats, the doctors know which charge nurses are adept at getting the team back on track.

"Honest disagreement is often a sign of good progress." — *Gandhi, Indian leader*

Be Prepared

As charge nurse you have to be prepared to handle conflict. It is an inevitable by-product of the intense human interaction in a busy patient care unit. Conflict is good in that it is a symptom of people really caring about what they do. Unfortunately, conflict can take the focus off the first priority—patient care.

Learning to manage conflict is one of the more demanding tasks that you must address as a charge nurse. It is stressful but, if you do it well, it can be empowering. Your confidence will grow and, as a result of your actions, members of the team may experience personal growth.

"A hero is no braver than an ordinary man, but he is brave five minutes longer." — *Ralph Waldo Emerson, author, poet, and philosopher*

Personal Lessons

Reflections

Reflect on your favorite supervisor
* How does this person handle conflict?
* What specific personal attributes help this supervisor resolve conflicts?
* Which of the quotes in this chapter would best describe this person's approach to work?

Reflect on yourself
* How do you manage conflict at work?
* Do you avoid? Accommodate? Collaborate? Force? Compromise?
* Do you lash out? Withdraw? Avoid? Collaborate? Stay calm?
* What are your buttons or triggers?
* How do you respond when these buttons are pushed?
* Do you find yourself getting involved in other peoples' conflicts?

Things to Remember

* Before you can help others through conflict, you need to be aware of how you manage conflict. In other words, you need to be self-aware about your ways of working through conflict. You must first be in tune with yourself before you can lead others effectively.
* The most difficult type of conflict to resolve is *interpersonal. Interpersonal* conflicts are often about

differences in values, issues or personality. They are often not about the current issue.

- *Situational* conflicts are usually temporary and exist in the moment. *Situational* conflicts often have to do with limited resources or incompatible priorities.
- As charge nurse you have to be prepared to manage conflict. It is an inevitable by-product of the intense human interaction inherent in a busy patient care unit.

Case Study—Dennis

At County Medical when an RN "calls off," other nurses have to cover the shift to care for the patients. Dennis, RN, is a good technical nurse, but he is a complainer. He consistently whines, regardless of who is in earshot. A unit has had three nurses call off and Dennis is asked to "float" to that unit. Upon arrival at the other unit, Sofia (charge nurse) greets Dennis saying, "We're glad to have you as part of our team today. We like having people from other units help us."

Dennis answers, "This isn't what I was hired to do. I'm only here because I have to be." Sofia ignores this and explains how the unit operates; however, through the entire orientation, Dennis' negative outlook continues. This starts getting on Sofia's nerves, but she does not confront the behavior.

As the day goes on, others on the unit begin noticing Dennis' attitude, including one patient's family member who mentions it to a doctor who tells Sofia. With so much going on, Sofia does not take time to deal with his behavior.

It is five hours into the shift, and Dennis has now offended three RNs. Sofia is at her limit. Two nurses have asked Sofia to take care of the issue. The unit is buzzing with drama, and the only one unaware of this is Dennis.

Review Questions:

- What is Sofia's next course of action?

- How does she resolve the conflict?
- How could all of this play out? After all, Sofia does not have any formal power over Dennis.
- What do you think?

Resources & References

Five Ways to Cope With Negative Colleagues
by Gary S. Topchik, *Managing Workplace Negativity*

People demonstrate their negative attitudes in many different ways. You can learn how to handle each one, but there are some general coping strategies.

Recognize that an attitude problem exists. The first step is to recognize that someone is expressing negativity in the workplace. Do not ignore it if it is affecting that person's performance, your performance, the performance of others or relationships with your clients or customers.

- Acknowledge any underlying causes for the negative attitude. As we know, negativity has many causes. The factors could include personal problems, work-related stress, a difficult boss, job insecurity, loss of loyalty, lack of growth or advancement opportunities and so forth. It helps to get the person to see the causes for his or her negativity. Ask non-threatening questions of colleagues like, "You look stressed. Can I help?" It is also important to recognize that what is causing the negativity is often justified and that the negativist has the right to feel that way.
- Help the person take responsibility. It is ultimately the responsibility of the negative person to change his or her negative attitude and behaviors at work. Even though the person may have every right to feel the way he or she does, it is still not appropriate for the workplace. As a team member or boss, you need to help your colleague recognize this and have him or her take ownership.

Consider addressing the problem privately with the person in a way that demonstrates concern for both their problems and the well-being of the team.

- Replace negative, inappropriate reactions with different, more acceptable ones. Even though we just said that it is the job of a negativist to change his or her actions, you may need to help. The person may not know what to do differently to come across as more positive. It will often be up to you to specify exactly what that is. You can suggest that people aren't aware of the person's great qualities or that his contributions are being eclipsed by negative behavior.
- Instill positive attitudes in others. Be the role model for your negativists through your actions and behaviors. You can prevent their negativity by instilling in them the positivist bug. If you do that, they may never catch the negativity virus again.
- Most of all, it's important to start a dialogue with difficult colleagues so issues can be addressed.

Reprinted with permission

Additional Resources

- *The Eight Essential Steps to Conflict Resolution: Preserving Relationships at Work, at Home, and in the Community* by Dudley Weeks
- *Managing Workplace Negativity* by Gary S. Topchik
- *Getting to Yes: Negotiating Agreement Without Giving In* by Roger Fisher, William L. Ury, and Bruce Patton
- *Crucial Conversations: Tools for Talking When Stakes Are High* by Kerry Patterson, Joseph Grenny, Ron McMillan, and Al Switzler

Stewart, K. (2003). *A Portable Mentor for Organizational Leaders.* Portsmouth, Ohio: SOMCPress, Inc.

Topchik, G. (2001). Five ways to cope with negative colleagues. *ivillage.com.* Retrieved December 13, 2103 from www.ivillage.com/5-ways-cope-negative-colleagues-0/4-a-283450.

Chapter Ten
Facilitating Change

The fact that few people enjoy changes at work is curious since everything changes all the time. We change. The people around us change. The seasons change. Life is full of change.

Many changes take place naturally. Things change without us taking much notice and certainly without our involvement or manipulation. We grow older. The trees grow taller. A favorite restaurant changes its menu.

We initiate and participate in many changes. We educate ourselves, find partners, have children and buy houses, cars and clothes. These are positive changes which we call "progress." However, at times we are unwilling participants in changes that we perceive as negative because they are emotionally or financially draining, and because they are beyond our control. They make us feel powerless. For example, family members lose their jobs, cars break down and so forth.

In fact, very little remains constant or stable in our lives. Every change requires us to regain our personal sense of balance and well-being. Depending on the effect of the change we are experiencing, the adjustment may be monumental or minimal.

"The combination of cultures that resist change and managers who have not been taught how to create change is lethal." — *John P. Kotter, author*

Change is Stressful

Because change can be stressful, we try to avoid the disruption whenever we feel that it is unnecessary, forced or harmful. Each of us has only so much capacity for stress and, as we mature, we know when we are near the point of painful imbalance. If the change we face seems more like an irritant than a positive, we fight against it.

When change is happening in our workplace it becomes more complex. Some people adapt well to change and easily roll with the ever-present adjustments. Others feel tired, frightened, angry, stupid and/or incompetent. At times, these feelings are manifested in the following behaviors: negativity, sarcasm, low energy and apathy. Of course, these behaviors take the joy out of what could be a positive and hopeful adjustment. So what can you do as the leader?

"Change means movement. Movement means friction. Only in the frictionless vacuum of a nonexistent abstract world can movement or change occur without that abrasive friction of conflict."—*Saul Alinsky, political activist*

Coping with Change

Understanding that everyone goes through a personal process of adjustment when faced with change is helpful. During my orientation period (Cathy) as a brand-new registered nurse, a revised form was introduced that changed the way we documented the care of patients with diabetes. I remember thinking "I am really going to like this job when they stop changing things." Little did I know that today change is inherent in health care. The good part is that, usually, innovations and refinements are aimed at improving our ability to care for patients. Knowing this makes change more bearable.

We know that in health care many improvements and updates are to come. Therefore, to find the workplace personally fulfilling, a nurse must learn to embrace change. Further, to be an effective charge nurse, it is necessary to become a *change agent*—the person leading change.

"Leadership is a relationship, founded on trust and confidence. Without trust and confidence, people don't take risks. Without

risks, there's no change. Without change, organizations and movements die." — *Jim Kouzes and Barry Posner, authors*

A Theory of Change

In 1962, Everett Rogers published the book *Diffusion of Innovations*. Some of you may have seen this concept mentioned in Simon Sinek's TED Talk, *How Great Leaders Inspire Action*. Rogers' studies showed that when people are faced with the introduction of innovations in the workplace, they fall into five categories: *innovators, early adopters, early majority, late majority and laggards*.

Innovators and *early adopters* make up roughly 17 percent of the workforce. These people embrace change and make it part of their daily routine. They understand the positive qualities and the performance improvement embedded in change and find change compatible with their existing values, past experiences and needs. They do not find change overly complex to understand and use. These people apply themselves to learning how to implement the change and they move on.

"It's not the strongest of the species that survives, nor the most intelligent. It is the one that is most adaptable to change."
— *Charles Darwin, British naturalist*

The three remaining categories, early and late majority and laggards, make up roughly 83 percent of the workforce. These people resist change on some level. They prefer to observe others incorporating change. They watch for visible results and need proof that change is worth the effort. Likewise, they want someone else to engage in a trial application before they invest themselves and may engage in verbal behavior that casts dispersions and doubts on innovation. Their behavior may even slow the transition from old to new.

Knowing this theory is helpful when you are a charge nurse. Think about which category best represents you and those on your unit. You are in a key position to be a change agent. The good news about Rogers' theory is that the innovators and early adopters can have a positive and powerful effect upon those who find change less comfortable.

Adopting this theory of change may make it easier for you to be an effective change agent. You can have a more positive influence on your coworkers when you understand their coping mechanisms.

"Change is the law of life. And those who look only to the past or present are certain to miss the future." — *John Fitzgerald Kennedy, 35th President of the United States*

Be an Effective Change Agent

Being a change agent requires you to be a role model for others. Be the change. Embrace it. Be flexible, agile and positive. Keep trying until you "get it." Learn everything you can and help others to learn. Talk about the positive reasons for the change and lead others through the process. Relate the change to *improved patient care*—this mantra is the common ground. When people are placing negative energy into resisting change, they are not placing positive energy into patient care. They are concentrating on the wrong thing. *They are thinking more about themselves than the patient.*

"God grant me the serenity to accept the things I cannot change, the courage to change the things I can, and the wisdom to know the difference." — *Reinhold Niebuhr, theologian*

Approach the adoption of change as a team. Teams are stronger than individuals. Be supportive of one another. Openly discussing the effect of the change is helpful, especially for those who resist it. People who are skeptical about change feel better when they realize they are not alone. Hearing about the approaches that have worked for others is encouraging. Doubters begin to relax when they hear that teammates have also experienced frustrations and are beginning to overcome those feelings. The trick is to keep these conversations positive. Foster and reinforce a positive culture that embraces change.

111

It is a good idea to become involved in committees and task forces that are developing innovations and changes. Let your supervisor know that you are interested in doing so. These work groups need the help of front-line nurses. The designers of change benefit from nursing input to make innovations fit with reality. Lacking the right information, the work groups may inadvertently create a gap between the planned change and essential approaches to care delivery. Your involvement as a frontline caregiver is invaluable.

People change what they do less because they are given analysis that shifts their thinking than because they are shown a truth that influences their feelings." — *John P. Kotter, author*

The Reality of Change

It is important to unscramble the *myth* of change from the *reality* of change, and to interpret this for the *late majority* and *laggards*. A marketing spin is often associated with change initiatives. Front line employees are told that the changes will make their work "better for the patient, the nurse and the physician." These messages are designed to achieve "buy-in." The problem with this approach is that it skips over the implementation phase, the learning curve and the "working-the-bumps-out" part of any change. Not only do leaders often omit any mention of this phase, but also they imply that implementation will be easy and seamless. In reality, the implementation phase is often difficult and fraught with challenges. The new technology may be disruptive, hard to use and at first, take longer. As a result, tempers flare and impatience reigns. Admitting this to one another and acknowledging it as a normal part of implementing change helps one another cope.

"Leaders are visionaries with a poorly developed sense of fear and no concept of the odds against them. They make the impossible happen." — *Dr. Robert Jarvik, American cardiac surgeon*

As a champion of change it is important for you to be aware that change implementation usually has two purposes: one is to *alter the manner* in which we do things (e.g., a new form, upgrading technology) and the second is to *improve our processes and outcomes* (e.g., embedding Evidence-Based Practice approaches into the care of patients). Therefore, we are often asked to learn two new concepts, not one. In a sense, the first is mechanical and the second is cognitive. The ease of implementing changes aimed at improving patient care is directly related to the gap between the old way and the new. The larger the gap, the longer the change will take, and the harder it will be to sustain. Can you think of an example of this in your own organization?

"Habits, values and attitudes, even dysfunctional ones, are part of one's identity. To change the way people see and do things is to challenge how they define themselves." — *Ronald Heifetz & Marty Linsky, authors*

Personal Lessons

Reflections

- What changes have you witnessed in your area?
- Of the ones that failed, what happened? Of the ones that succeeded, why were they successful?
- What are some of the major challenges your organization faces when implementing a change?
- What are some of the major challenges your unit faces when implementing a change?
- Which one are you: an innovator, an early adopter, an early majority, a late majority, or a laggard? Which one do you want to be?
- What are some of the major challenges *you* face when implementing a change?
- What can you do to help facilitate change on your unit?
- What challenges will you face?
- What resources can you tap to help you along?
- Who in the organization can help you along?

- There is very little that remains constant or stable in our lives. Every change requires us to regain our personal sense of balance and well-being.
- Everett Rogers' *Diffusion of Innovation Theory* suggests that when people are faced with the introduction of innovations in the work place they fall into five categories: *innovators, early adopters, early majority, late majority and laggards.*
- Behaviors, training, accountability and rewards must all be part of your plan. If they are not, it will likely fall short.
- The implementation of change usually has two purposes. The first is to *alter the manner* in which we do things and the second is to *improve our processes and outcomes.* Therefore, we are often asked to learn two new concepts, not one.

Case Study—Scripting

You are the charge nurse during day shift on a pediatric unit. Your supervisor has told you that administration would like you to implement *scripting*. Nurses are to use scripted messages when they speak with patients. For instance, when you are about to leave a patient's room you are to say, "Is there anything else I can do for you?" You have been told that this approach improves customer satisfaction and makes life easier for nurses. Hmmm…you do not see how this is will make your life *any* easier. There are already a million things going on.

Regardless, your supervisor asks you to implement the scripting on your shift. You know those around you will be resistant because this feels like another "flavor of the month." To make it worse, you are not even sure you agree with the new request.

Review Questions:

- How do you go about implementing this change?

- What resources are at your disposal to help in making this adjustment?
- How will your demeanor and attitude toward the change impact its successful implementation?
- What is your plan of action?

Resources & References

Terms & Acronyms

- **Change Agent**—Someone who knows and understands the dynamics that facilitate or hinder change. Someone who acts to alter human capability or organizational systems to a higher degree of output or self-actualization.
- **Change Initiative**—an initiative with the specific purpose of changing organizational norms and behaviors.
- **Change Management**—the act of managing the process of organizational change. Change management is often associated with a plan of action designed in advance.

Additional Resources

- *Leading Change* by John P. Kotter
- *The Heart of Change: Real-Life Stories of How People Change Their Organizations* by John P. Kotter & Dan S. Cohen
- *The Leadership Challenge* by Jim Kouzes & Barry Posner
- *Leadership on the Line* by Ron Heifetz & Marty Linsky

References

Rogers, E. M. (1962). *Diffusion of innovations*. New York: Simon & Schuster, Inc.

Chapter Eleven
Clarifying Expectations/Effective Communication

One day when I (Cathy) was the charge nurse, I asked the bedside nurse for an update on the discharge plan for one of our patients who was to go home the next day. I was dismayed when she said, "He went home an hour ago. Did you say discharge *tomorrow*!? I thought you said discharge *today*. Should I call the doctor and tell him the patient has already been discharged?"

This is not what you want to hear from a member of your team and this is the hard way to learn the importance of clarifying expectations. Of course, this example is an extreme one in which many concepts of safe practice and nursing judgment have been violated. But it makes the point about how terribly wrong things can go when just one word is misunderstood. Communicating clearly and clarifying one another's expectations is extremely important in the care of patients. Further, it saves everyone a lot of precious time.

This chapter is about communication—the giving and receiving of information. Communication that is clear and mutually agreed upon by all parties involved is essential to the safety and well-being of patients. We have touched on the topic of stakeholders who depend upon you for communication and information. In fact communication is a common thread that weaves throughout the book and the topic of leadership. Giving some thought to what is expected of you and others may help you to succeed in your leadership role.

"The quality of our expectations determines the quality of our actions." — *Andre Godin, French socialist*

There are many parties that depend on you to be clear and accurate in your communication of information. It may help to think about the expectations of all parties. The first step in clarifying expectations is to be aware of who the stakeholders are. Here is a partial list of possible stakeholders that you interface with on a regular basis, either directly or indirectly:

- patients and their significant others
- nursing team, physicians and other direct caregivers
- extended team—support people and departments
- your supervisor
- the organization that employs you
- care partners external to the organization (e.g., home care nurses)
- external regulatory bodies (e.g., State Nursing Board, JCAHO and the Department of Health)
- you (yes, you interact with yourself in reflection and as you make decisions)

It is sobering to realize how many people and organizations are dependent upon clear communication with each other. To provide safe and effective nursing care, it is important to know what is expected of each other. Some knowledge of the expectations of yourself and others will help you to be more effective in your work.

You know that ultimately all stakeholders expect you to do what is right for the patient(s). This is a simple maxim, but, in the complexity of daily care, it is not so simple to figure out what *is* right for the patient. The patient, their significant others and every professional involved in the patient's care may have different opinions. Each has individual biases, unique experiences, professional education/knowledge, other priorities, personal desires and motivations. The expectations of indirect and external stakeholders are often time consuming and may seem irrelevant to the immediacy of patient care. As charge nurse, you must consider the input and the expectations of all parties. Then, acting as the patient's advocate and leader of the team, you must make the best possible decisions…often quickly.

"A master can tell you what he expects of you. A teacher, though, awakens your own expectations." — *Patricia Neal, actress*

Clarify Expectations of Yourself

Returning to the list above, you will note that one of the stakeholders to consider is you. To keep the patient at the top of the list, you must first understand yourself. Therefore, it is a good idea to clarify the expectations you have for yourself. Your expectations likely include: giving the best care possible to each patient, having a collegial relationship with your peers, improving and learning each day, having fun, being a role model, impressing your supervisor, being strong, feeling fulfilled, knowing you are making a positive difference in the lives of others, being trusted and respected, and being accountable and responsible. Reflecting upon what you expect from yourself is a good exercise. Doing so keeps you grounded in a deep understanding of the greater meaning of your work. Likewise, personal reflection may reveal areas of nonalignment between your own expectations and those of others. Therein lies the path to further growth and learning.

As a leader you must be clear on the expectations of your supervisor and the organization. *This is the roadmap to success* in your current context. It can be difficult to find time for conversations of this nature. Don't hesitate to request a meeting with your supervisor to seek feedback and clarification about what is expected of you. You deserve to find out how you are doing from the supervisor's perspective and your supervisor owes this to you as well.

Other sources to help you clarify expectations are your position description, orientation, competency testing, in-services and policies and procedures. However, the most personal and valuable source may be your peers and mentors. Ask what you are doing right. Ask what aspects of your practice need improvement. See how the responses fit with your own perceptions. This reflective process will make you a better charge nurse.

Ultimately, you will feel as though you are part of the "bigger picture" if you know what the organization expects of you. Some basic questions may include:

- What does our mission and vision statement communicate?
- What is in our strategic plan?
- What action plans are applicable to our nursing unit?
- What indicators are being measured for performance improvement or by the quality assurance department?
- What are the unit's and organization's goals for performance?
- How does my daily practice help achieve these goals?

"Winners make a habit of manufacturing their own positive expectations in advance of the event." — *Brian Tracy, leadership author*

The Key to Clarifying Expectations: Communication

The nitty-gritty of nursing practice rests in the communication and clarification of expectations with patients, significant others, the nursing team and physicians. As you know, clarifying expectations is not as easy as it sounds because many factors implicit to health care have a negative effect on the clarity and thoroughness of communication. You need to be aware of them. These factors may include: stress, frustration, a lack of time, competing commitments, anxiety, anger, cultural differences, pain, illness and multi-tasking. It takes time to clarify expectations with each other, but it saves time in the end…and it is much more therapeutic for the patient.

It is always a good idea to remember that if people do not know what is expected of them, there is no way to hold them accountable for their actions or lack thereof.

"Set your expectations high; find men and women whose integrity and values you respect; get their agreement on a

course of action; and give them your ultimate trust."—*John Akers, former IBM chairman*

In your role as charge nurse you need to clarify expectations with each of your stakeholders countless times each shift. Speak clearly. State the facts and, in a kind way, ask people if they understand what you've said. Listen to their responses and observe their non-verbal behaviors. If there is confusion or disagreement, stop and discuss until there is consensus. Likewise, listen to the other person's point of view. Stephen Covey's fifth principle in *The 7 Habits of Highly Effective People* is: "Seek first to understand, then to be understood."

If you are taking directives from someone else (e.g., orders from a physician), repeat them. Ask questions if there are confusing or conflicting messages. Make sure expectations are clarified. As you know, this is sometimes difficult if the messenger is in a hurry or in an impatient state of mind. However, as the patient's advocate, you have to work through these barriers and clarify the expectations. In the end, it will save everyone time and the patients will get the care they deserve and require. Repeating verbal orders to the initiator is not only wise and safe, but also required by JCAHO.

"If you paint in your mind a picture of bright and happy expectations, you put yourself into a condition conducive to your goal." — *Norman Vincent Peale, author and clergyman*

As the charge nurse, it may be your role at times to help patients and their significant others understand information that is confusing them. This is often not an easy or quick task. It requires time, listening, detective work, and facilitating communication among members of the healthcare team. There are many people who come in and out of a patient's room and to the patient, these caregivers do not all seem to be on the same page. If there are several physicians on the case, they may not be aware of what each other has said to the patient. The same is true of other caregivers. It gets even more complicated when there are several significant others who have heard mixed messages and perceive the situation in different ways. Trying your best to clarify expectations in these situations is critical. Patient-satisfaction survey results show that the nurse-patient relationship and nurse communication have the greatest impact on a patient's overall satisfaction. So even if it takes a long time and is difficult to do, it is worth it—well worth it—to listen to the questions and concerns of the patient and family and then to clarify, as much as you can, what the patient can expect from the healthcare team. You and your nursing team are the people closest to, and most trusted by, the patient. The positive effect you have in communicating with the patient goes a long way toward promoting healing and giving the patient a sense of well-being.

"Our limitations and successes will be based, most often, on our expectations for ourselves. What the mind dwells upon, the body acts upon." — *Denis Waitley, leadership author*

Personal Lessons

Things to Do

- Read the position description of a charge nurse for your facility.
- Know the expectations of your supervisor.
- Know the expectations of your co-workers.
- Know the expectations of the physicians.
- Know the expectations of external regulatory organizations such as JCAHO.
- Know the expectations of your patients and their significant others.
- Articulate what the above-mentioned people can expect from you.
- Know the mission, vision, goals and objectives of your organization.

- What is your plan for clarifying the above-mentioned expectations?
- What are some ways and resources to help you find answers to the statements in the "Things to Do" section?
- Who among your peers does a great job of setting expectations? Why are they successful?
- What happens when clear expectations are not part of the culture? How does this affect patient care?
- When was the last time *you* did not communicate clearly to one of the stakeholders mentioned in this chapter? What were the results?

Things to Remember

- "Take the needed time to work with individuals who are not meeting your expectations. It is important not only for you to communicate initially what you expect, but also if you see a consistent pattern that is not what you are looking for, take the time to adjust it. Don't ignore it and let it continue; if you do, you'll either be the one redoing the project or getting consistently frustrated."—Peggy L. McNamara
- It is a good idea to clarify the expectations you have for yourself. Your expectations probably include: giving the best care possible to each patient, having a collegial relationship with your peers, improving and learning each day, having fun, being a role model, impressing your supervisor, being strong, feeling fulfilled, knowing you are making a positive difference in the lives of others, being trusted and respected and being accountable and responsible.
- In all of your interactions, remember Stephen Covey's fifth principle in *The 7 Habits of Highly Effective People*: Seek first to understand, then to be understood.
- As charge nurse, it may be your role to help patients and their significant others understand information that is confusing. Often, this is not a quick or easy task. Doing so

requires time, listening, detective work and, sometimes, facilitating communication among members of the healthcare team.

Case Study—County Medical Center

You are relatively new to County Medical Center (CMC) and have been assigned to be in charge on the late shift in the ICU. You work nights and often feel somewhat disconnected from the "daytime" medical center.

However, you are excited to be in this new role and want to make a difference. You have always known that your strengths lie in your people skills. You have an ability to work with people of all kinds and not get caught up in some of the "catty" aspects of the unit. You are unfamiliar with the role of charge nurse, and by no means do you have a grasp of the many administrative or managerial policies and procedures.

Although the players change each night, your team usually is comprised of the following individuals:

- Sandy Johnson, RN, MSN, has been in the ICU for 23 years. She knows everything there is to know about the ICU and is very involved; however, she is extremely overbearing and will tell *everyone* her thoughts on *everything*. She is not happy that you are the charge nurse.
- Maria Sandoza, RN, and Cheri O'Malley, RN, BSN, pretty much keep to themselves. They always want to go on break at the same time and do their assignments together, but are not willing to do much beyond that. They tend to feed the rumor mill but, more often than not, they can be counted on to complete their assignments.
- Jenny Peters, RN, BSN, and David Rae, RN, have been with CMC for 12 years. Their families come first and often they arrive late because of family commitments. They are good employees, but rarely get to work on time and they often take frequent breaks.

- Wenyan Wen, RN, is the nicest person to be around and is very agreeable; however, her mistakes are abundant. It seems that you spend a good portion of your time cleaning up after Wenyan or listening to others complain about her inadequacies.
- Jessica Walters, RN, and Molly Mathers, RN, BSN, have been at odds with each other for years. They are constantly in conflict and, when not talking about each other, they are talking about how inadequate everyone else is. They each run with some of the above-mentioned individuals and often their differences boil over into the two cliques. Both Jessica and Molly like to tell others about their issues with the other. Everyone is tired of it.
- Ben Swartz, RN, Mary Tharp, RN, and Dana Ryszetnyk, RN are your closest friends on the unit. They have stuck with you through thick and thin. They always keep you "in the loop." None of them is perfect and at times they gossip. They have punctuality issues but you feel strongly that they are good people and are "here for the patient."
- Wanda Wallingford is the unit secretary and has been with the organization for 30 years. She is kind, compassionate and trustworthy. She seems to be the glue that holds the unit together.
- Three EMTs work on your unit and each has a bit of an attitude. Martin Cobb can be lazy and always has to be told what to do. Jud Horras is very competent, but has personality conflicts with many people on the unit. Mike McRee does not always follow the rules and can be a bit dramatic—often leaving before fulfilling all of his duties.

Review Questions:

- Based on the content of this chapter, what are five things you can do to promote teamwork on the unit?
- What are five things you can do to improve communication on the unit?
- What are five ways to provide feedback to your team members with performance issues? How do you set

expectations with everyone? What should those expectations be?

- What are five things you need to keep in mind from Chapter One as you begin working with your unit?
- What resources/tools may assist you in providing excellent care to the patients?

Resources & References

Terms & Acronyms

- **Performance Improvement (PI), Quality Assurance (QA), Total Quality Management (TQM)**—These are comprehensive and structured approaches that seek to improve the quality of care and services through ongoing refinements in response to continuous measurement and feedback. All of these approaches focus on improving the systems around you so that outcomes are improved.

Additional Resources

- *Managing Patient Expectations: The Art of Finding and Keeping Loyal Patients* by Susan Keane Baker
- *Managing Expectations* by Naomi Karten
- *Exceptional Customer Service: Going Beyond Your Good Service to Exceed the Customer's Expectation* by Lisa Ford, *et al.*

References

Covey, S. (1989). *The 7 habits of highly effective people.* New York: Simon & Schuster.

Chapter Twelve
Remember Your Mission

It seems like this would go without saying.

You are here for the patient. You are here to make sure the patient receives great care and, in your role as charge nurse, you do much of this through other people. Therefore, you are here to be the best leader possible. Through your influence and guidance, your mission is to motivate the healthcare team to provide the very best health care possible.

While it may seem obvious, reminding yourself that you are here for the patient is essential. The team must remember this fact as well. Healthcare organizations are so busy, stressful, fast-paced and full of competing priorities that sometimes the reason for our work becomes obscured. We are only human and yet our work demands us—and we demand of ourselves—to be superhuman. It can be easy to get off track, discouraged, frustrated and overwhelmed.

"The sheer act of love transcends the outcome." — *Mother Teresa, spiritual leader*

One day a physician called me (Cathy) from his car. It was early in the morning and he was visiting all of his patients in various hospitals before he opened for office hours. He was trying to be in several places at once. He asked if I would bring all of his patients' charts to the front desk so that he could make entries in them without having to actually make rounds. *He had forgotten his mission.* We talked for a few minutes about how much his patients were looking forward to seeing him. He realized without having to say it out loud how far he had strayed from his purpose. He made rounds. He got back on track.

"It is the nature of man to rise to greatness if greatness is expected of him." — *John Steinbeck, author*

Here is another example. When I served as a hospital executive, departments developed goals and action plans each year. It was my task to review the plans to make sure they supported the mission and goals of the organization. In reviewing the plan of a support department an omission was found. The employees in this department were not responsible for direct patient care; however, through their daily work they supported direct patient caregivers. As I read their goals and action plans, I realized that nowhere in the document had they used the word *patient*. It was evident that serving the patient was implied, but it was not directly stated. I sent the document back for revision. It was a good department. They did their work well, but I felt it was important that they remember their mission by including the word *"patient"* in their annual plan of work.

"Technological improvements do not do away with the importance of having that link with an individual, that response from another being, which is what nursing perhaps defines most clearly." — *Queen Elizabeth II of England*

Staying on Track

Now and then in the course of your personal and professional life, it is good to stop and reflect upon where you are in relation to your mission. Why did you become a nurse in the first place? Why did you choose this profession as your life's work? Do you remember your first clinical rotation? Do you remember that feeling of eagerness to be a nurse someday? Do you remember the day you passed your state board examination? Do you remember your first day on the job? Can you believe how much you have learned and grown since then?

It is good to reflect upon how far you have come and where you are going. Thinking about where you are today compared with where you aspire to be is a good mental exercise. It is motivating to have goals and to work toward them Then, once they are achieved, to set new goals that allow you to grow and stretch even more. You will find strength and inspiration in understanding the gap between the realities of who you are now and the vision of who you want to be.

"Nurses know how to listen, how to reach out, how to respect."
— *Comelio Sommaruga, President, International Committee of the Red Cross*

Your Personal Mission Statement

One of the final topics we will explore is that of mission. In a sense, everything should flow from your personal mission. And, if your mission is strong, it will serve as your north star. Mentoring, patient safety, patient satisfactions, addressing conflict and leadership will all flow from the soul of your being.

You are the only one who knows your personal mission. Take some time to think about it. What is your mission each day? Each year? For your life? Writing down your personal mission, values and goals is a worthwhile exercise. Doing so helps you think about what is important to you and what you want to accomplish. Read it once a month and ask yourself: Am I on track? Am I proud of the person I see in the mirror? Are the people I care about proud of me? Am I the kind of adult I dreamed about being when I was a child? Am I living up to my potential? Am I being all I can be? Am I taking care of myself?

A written mission or vision is a powerful tool. A shortened (six to ten word) version can become a daily mantra to help you stay on track. As nurses we have a tendency to reflect negatively upon our work—we dwell on what we did not get done, and what we should have done. Replace those self-deprecating thoughts with positive thoughts "I did a lot of good today. I made a positive difference in many lives."

It is your mission, too, to represent the nursing profession. Now and then, a poll is conducted to survey the public's perception of various professional groups. Almost always, nurses come out at the very top as being honest, ethical and trusted (Hitti, 2004). The public has a very high opinion of nurses. It is the responsibility of each of us to live up to that reputation. We know from patient satisfaction surveys that nurses are valued highly for their ability to balance competency and technical know-how with caring and compassion. Nurses are valued for their ability to develop relationships with patients through listening, explaining and the demonstration of caring.

Mission Defined

A personal mission statement will answer three primary questions:

- What is the purpose of my life?
- What values do I hold dear?
- What do those values look like in action?

An acute sense of your *values in action* is the most important piece. Once your personal mission statement is written, you need to reflect on how you are doing. You need to revisit it when you are down. You need to share it with others so they can help you. You need to make it a part of your life. Otherwise, it will be words on paper, in a notebook on a shelf, and not "living" and guiding you.

Another way to think about your personal mission is to imagine the following scenario: you are retiring tomorrow and the nurses on your unit are each responsible for saying something about you in front of the group. They have taken truth serum and will offer their honest thoughts. If this were in fact tomorrow, what would they say? What are their perceptions of you and your work? Would they see you as you see yourself as outlined in your mission statement? Answering these questions in an honest fashion can give you a rough idea of how your role as charge nurse aligns with your personal mission statement.

Conclusion

In the beginning of this book we defined personal mission as a "pre-established and often self-imposed objective or purpose." To us, each of you reading this book exemplifies a noble purpose. A person with a mission that is so very important. Thank you.

Nursing is a complex profession. It requires the qualities sought after by the lion, the scarecrow and the tin man in *The Wizard of Oz*. Courage, Brains and Heart. Risk-taking, critical thinking, and caring. Thank you for taking on this challenge and doing your best possible work. Doing so will improve you, your staff, your unit and patient experience.

To conclude this book, we will end where we began. We hope that as you read it again, the words have a little more meaning than they did before. Likewise we hope you feel more confident in your knowledge, skills and abilities to successfully take on this very important role. We hope that you are proud to represent what Robert Frost speaks of in his poem for his nurse, Janet Forbes:

"I met you on a cloudy and dark day and when you smiled and spoke the room was filled with sunshine. The way you smiled at me has given my heart a change of mood and saved some part of a day I had rued."

You are the symbol of hope, comfort and caring.

References

Frost, R. (n.d.). *Miss Forbes*. Quoted in an article by Klein, J. (2002). Teaching palliative care and education. *Oncology Times*, *24*(12), 79-80.

Hitti, M. (2004). Nurses top list for honesty. Webmd.com. Retrieved December 24, 2013 from women.webmd.com/news/20041208/nurses-top-list-for-honesty.

About the Authors

Cathy Leary

Cathy is a Registered Nurse with licensure in the state of Ohio. She holds a BA in Psychology, an MS in Nursing Administration and a Nursing Diploma. She has extensive experience in the acute care setting as a bedside nurse, a nurse administrator and a hospital executive. She has worked across the country as a healthcare consultant. Cathy is trained as a Malcolm Baldrige Examiner. Experience has taught her that charge nurses and other nurse leaders are the key to high quality health care.

Scott J. Allen

Scott J. Allen, Ph.D., is associate professor of management at John Carroll University. His research interests include leadership development and emotionally intelligent leadership. Scott serves as an associate editor for the *Journal of Management Education* and is the co-author of *The Little Book of Leadership Development* and *Emotionally Intelligent Leadership: A Guide for College Students.* In addition to teaching and writing, Scott conducts workshops, leads retreats and consults across industries. Scott is a member of The Association of Leadership Educators, The Academy of Management, OBTS Teaching Society for Management Educators and serves on the boards of the International Leadership Association and Beta Theta Pi Fraternity.

Contact the Authors

We would love to hear from you! How can we improve this book? What stories would you like to share? What should we include in future editions?

Cathy Leary and Scott J. Allen may be contacted for inquires, speaking engagements, workshops and interviews as follows:

Cathy Leary, R.N.
Phone: 216-406-6245
Email: cathyleary1@netscape.net

Scott J. Allen, Ph.D.
Phone: 216-224-7072
Email: scott@cldmail.com

Order Information

To order copies of this publication, contact BookMasters at:

Phone: 800-537-6727
Fax: 419-281-0200
Email: orders@bookmasters.com
Web: www.atlasbooks.com
Mail: Bookmasters Inc.
        30 Amberwood Parkway
        Ashland, Ohio 44805